HANDBOOK FOR
INFECTIOUS DISEASE
MANAGEMENT

Cornelis A. Kolff, MD, MPH

Assistant Clinical Instructor in Pediatrics
University of Washington

National Health Service Corps Physician
Sea Mar Community Health Center
Seattle, Washington

Ramón C. Sánchez, MD, MPH

Assistant Professor of Health Services–Community Medicine
Adjunct Assistant Professor of Family Medicine
University of Washington
Seattle, Washington

ADDISON-WESLEY PUBLISHING COMPANY
Medical/Nursing Division

Menlo Park, California • Reading, Massachusetts
London • Amsterdam • Don Mills, Ontario • Sydney

Library of Congress Cataloging in Publication Data

Kolff, Cornelis A. 1945–
  Handbook for infectious disease management.
  Bibliography: p.
  Includes index.
  1. Communicable diseases. I. Sánchez,
Ramón C., 1946– joint author. II. Title.
RC111.K64 616.9.   79-11377
ISBN 0-201-03892-7

ABCDEFGHIJ-HA-782109

Addison-Wesley Publishing Company
Medical/Nursing Division
2725 Sand Hill Road
Menlo Park, California 94025

PREFACE

The purpose of this book is to present clinically useful information on infectious diseases in a manner that is both convenient for quick reference and graphic for instruction. This book is not meant to be a comprehensive, definitive reference. Rather, it is meant to be a description of an approach, a listing of critical information, and an outline of some guidelines that may prove useful in

- Making a diagnosis
- Formulating a treatment plan
- Preventing the spread

of infectious diseases in a primary-care setting.

This book is intended for those learning, practicing, and teaching the primary care of patients with infectious diseases:

- Physicians
- Nurses
- Students

Different sections of this book will be particularly useful at different times. A physician prescribing antimicrobials may find Chapter 3 the most useful; a nurse involved in home care, Chapter 7, and a student learning decision-making, the algorithms in Chapter 2. We feel that it is helpful for all three groups to have ready access to each other's source of information in one book.

During our combined training and experience in public health, epidemiology, pediatrics, family medicine, and now primary care, we became convinced there was a better way of packaging the answers to the most commonly asked questions on infectious diseases. Depending on the

- Specialists consulted
- Local geographic preferences
- Microbial resistance patterns

and hosts of other factors, there are often various acceptable methods of handling infectious disease problems. We have tried to present at least one useful approach from a primary care perspective.

▶ **ACKNOWLEDGMENTS**

We are sincerely grateful to the following individuals for their ideas and assistance: Naomi Bock; Larry Corey, MD; Mickey Eisenberg, MD, MPH; Clarice Hargiss, RN; Carol Kirby; Mary Lampe; Judy Lew; Edgar Marcuse, MD, MPH; Karen McMasters; Mary Medina, MS; Henry Negrón, MD; George Ray, MD; José Rigau, MD; Fritz Schoenknecht, MD; Walter Stamm, MD; Steven Teutsch, MD; Yvonne Tso, RPh; Melanie Tyler; Marion Wagenaar.

The University of Washington, and particularly the Robert Wood Johnson Clinical Scholars Program, was most supportive during the preparation of this book.

CONTENTS

*Refer to the first page of these chapters for a detailed contents listing.

1

THE INITIAL APPROACH

CONTENTS

PERTINENT CONSIDERATIONS IN THE INITIAL APPROACH

▶ **DIAGNOSTIC**

- How sick, uncomfortable, and unstable is the patient?
- Where is the most probable primary source of infection based on symptoms and physical findings?
- What quick laboratory results are worth doing (gram stain, U/A, CBC, X ray, etc.)?
- Which category of infectious agent is suspected (bacterial, viral, fungal, parasitic, or other)?
- Which organisms are the most probable etiologic agents based on:
  - symptoms and physical findings
  - available laboratory data
  - age and past history of patient
  - sociodemographic information
  - known frequency of occurrence of specific pathogens in the primary site of involvement
- Which transport and/or culture media are most appropriate?
- Is definitive laboratory confirmation warranted? If so, what measures must be taken to obtain specimens (swabs, body fluid collection, biopsies)?

▶ **MANAGEMENT**

- Do special patient-handling procedures or isolation measures (like gloving, gowning, masking) need to be initiated?
- Should antimicrobial therapy be initiated prior to the isolation of the pathogen?
- Which antimicrobials are indicated for initial treatment, taking into account:
  - likely pathogens
  - efficacy of treatment
  - side effects
  - cost
  - patient comfort
  - route, frequency, and duration of treatment
- Can the patient be treated as an outpatient, or should he/she be hospitalized?
- What measures for monitoring patient response should be instigated, and what follow-up schedule will be most informative to the clinician and convenient for the patient?
- What information and reassurance must be related to the patient?
- Do measures for controlling the spread of the suspected disease include:
  - isolation
  - reporting
  - prophylaxis

INITIAL ANTIBIOTIC MANAGEMENT OF SELECTED
ACUTE INFECTIONS IF PATHOGENS ARE UNKNOWN

Often, because of cost-effectiveness concerns, limited laboratory information or other constraints, one is forced to make antibiotic therapy decisions that are based on limited information, rather than on conclusive conformitory data. *Decision making in the face of uncertainty is the art of medicine.* The following information is intended to assist the clinician in making better choices in the face of uncertainty. The recommendations presented are guidelines and may have to be modified by the severity of illness, the clinician's local experience, the patient's immune status, and various other factors.

Infection	Age	Usual Pathogens	Acceptable Initial Antibiotics If Pathogen Unknown
Abscess, Skin	All ages	*Staphylococcus aureus*	Penicillinase-resistant penicillin (e.g., cloxacillin) PO *or* erythromycin PO
Arthritis, Septic	0–2 months	*S. aureus* Streptococcus *Escherichia coli* Klebsiella *Neisseria gonorrhea*	Methicillin IV *plus* gentamicin IV
	2 months– 4 years	*Haemophilus influenzae* *S. aureus*	Methicillin IV *plus* ampicillin IV
	Over 4 years	*S. aureus*	Methicillin IV
	Adults	*N. gonorrhea*	Penicillin IV *or* IM
Cellulitis	All ages	*Streptococcus pyogenes* *S. aureus*	Penicillin PO *or* penicillinase-resistant penicillin PO
(Facial or peri- orbital)	Under 5 years	Also consider *H. influenza*	Ampicillin IV *plus* methicillin IV
Cervicitis (see Vaginitis)			
Conjunctivitis	Neonate	*Chlamydia trachomatis* *N. gonorrhea*	Topical sulfonamide 10% *or* *topical* tetracycline
	All ages	*S. aureus* *Streptococcus pneumoniae* *H. influenzae* *E. coli* Proteus spp	Topical sulfonamide

Infection	Age	Usual Pathogens	Acceptable Initial Antibiotics If Pathogen Unknown
Endocarditis, Bacterial	Child	Streptococcus spp Enterococcus	Penicillin IV *plus* gentamicin IV
	Adult (addict)	S. aureus Gram-negative organisms	Methicillin IV *plus* gentamicin IV
	Adult (non-addict)	Enterococcus Streptococcus spp	Penicillin *or* ampicillin IV *plus* gentamicin IV
Epiglottitis	Any age	H. influenzae	Chloramphenicol IV *or* ampicillin IV
Gastroenteritis*	Neonate	E. coli	Neomycin PO *or* colistin sulfate
	All ages	Shigella spp Salmonella spp	Ampicillin PO Chloramphenicol *or* ampicillin PO
		E. coli	Neomycin PO
Impetigo	All ages	Streptococcus spp S. aureus	Penicillin PO *or* IM *or* erythromycin PO *or* penicillinase-resistant penicillin PO
Mastitis	Adult	S. aureus	Penicillinase-resistant penicillin PO (e.g., cloxacillin)
Meningitis	Infants	Gram-negative enterics S. pyogenes Listeria	Ampicillin IV *plus* gentamicin *or* kanamycin IV, IT *or* chloramphenicol IV
	Children over 2 months	H. influenzae	Chloramphenicol IV *plus* ampicillin IV

*No treatment needed unless patient is toxic or bacteremia is suspected.

Infection	Age	Usual Pathogens	Acceptable Initial Antibiotics If Pathogen Unknown
Meningitis (cont.)	Young adults	H. influenzae N. meningitidis S. pneumoniae	Ampicillin IV
	Adults	N. meningitidis S. pneumoniae	Penicillin IV
Osteomyelitis	0–6 months	S. aureus Streptococcus spp E. coli Klebsiella	Methicillin IV plus gentamicin IV
	Over 6 months	S. aureus	Methicillin IV
Otitis Media	Neonate	Gram-negative enterics Group B streptococci	Ampicillin PO or IV
	0–5 years	H. influenzae S. pneumoniae S. pyogenes	Ampicillin PO or penicillin PO or IM and sulfisoxazole PO
	Over 5 years	S. pneumoniae S. pyogenes	Penicillin PO or IM or amoxicillin PO or ampicillin PO
Pelvic Inflammatory Disease	Adults	E. coli N. gonorrhea H. vaginalis Chlamydiae	Ampicillin PO or tetracycline PO or cephalosporin
Pharyngitis	Any age	S. pyogenes (Group A streptococci) N. gonorrhea C. diphtheriae	Penicillin PO or IM or erythromycin PO
Pneumonia	Neonate	S. aureus Pseudomonas aeruginosa	Methicillin IV plus gentamicin or kanamycin IV

Infection	Age	Usual Pathogens	Acceptable Initial Antibiotics If Pathogen Unknown
Pneumonia (Cont.)	Any age	*S. pneumoniae* *Mycoplasma pneumoniae* *Klebsiella pneumoniae* *S. aureus* *H. influenzae* *C. trachomatis*	Penicillin PO *or* cephalosporin PO *or* erythromycin PO
Prostatitis or Epididymitis	Adult	*N. gonorrhea* *S. aureus* Chlamydia spp	Co-Trimoxazole (Bactrim)
Sepsis	Neonate	Gram-negative enteric bacilli Group B streptococci Listeria *S. aureus*	Ampicillin IV *plus* gentamicin *or* kanamycin IV
	Child	*H. influenzae* *N. meningitidis*	Ampicillin *or* penicillin *or* methicillin IV *plus* gentamicin *or* chloramphenicol IV
	Child (with leukemia or cystic fibrosis)	*Ps. aeruginosa*	Carbenicillin IV *plus* gentamicin IV
	Adult	Gram-negative enteric bacilli	Penicillinase-resistant penicillin (*or* ampicillin *or* carbenicillin *or* cephalosporin) IV *plus* gentamicin *or* tobramycin IV
		Bacteroides	Chloramphenicol *or* clindamycin IV

Infection	Age	Usual Pathogens	Acceptable Initial Antibiotics If Pathogen Unknown
Sinusitis	Any age	S. pyogenes H. influenzae S. pneumoniae	Penicillin or amoxicillin or ampicillin or erythromycin or
		S. aureus	Penicillinase-resistant penicillin PO
Urinary Tract Infections	Neonate	Gram-negative enteric bacilli	Ampicillin PO plus gentamycin or kanamycin PO
	Any age	E. coli Klebsiella Proteus Pseudomonas Enterococcus S. aureus C. trachomatis	Sulfisoxazole PO or ampicillin PO
Vaginitis– Cervicitis	Any age	H. vaginalis	Triple sulfa vaginally or Ampicillin PO or Metronidazole PO
		Trichomonas vaginalis	Metronidazole PO
		C. albicans	Nystatin (vaginally)
		Chlamydia spp	Tetracycline PO
		N. gonorrhea	Penicillin IM
Urethritis (Male)	Any age with sexual activity	N. gonorrhea Chlamydia spp Mycoplasma spp	Tetracycline PO or erythromycin PO or Co-Trimoxazole (Bactrim)

LABORATORY TESTS USEFUL IN DIAGNOSING INFECTIONS

The choice of specific laboratory tests should be based on the following factors:

- The history and physical examination are frequently all that is necessary to establish a presumptive diagnosis. Starting therapeutic management without further confirmation is often warranted.
- The cost-benefit of all tests should be carefully considered.
  Costs include: patient discomfort, direct costs, inconvenience, time delay, risk of complications, and false positive or negative misdiagnosis.
  Benefits include: confirmation of the correct diagnosis and increase of reassurance for patient and provider.

NONSPECIFIC TESTS		
Test	*Normal Range*	*Abnormal Findings in Selected Diseases*
TOTAL WHITE BLOOD COUNT (WBC)	4000–12,000/mm^3 (up to 35,000 in newborns and 15,000 in 1-year olds)	↑ in most systemic infections
DIFFERENTIAL WBC		
• lymphs	25%–33%	↑ in many viral infections
• polys and bands (left shift)	Up to 60%	↑ in many bacterial infections
• monocytes	Up to 7%	↑ in mononucleosis
• eosinophils	Up to 600/mm^3	↑ in many parasitic infestations
SEDIMENTATION RATE	Men: 0–8 mm/hour Women: 0–15 mm/hour Children: 4–13 mm/hour	↑ in many bacterial infections

SEMI-SPECIFIC TESTS

Test	Normal Range	Abnormal Findings in Selected Diseases
URINE (clean, void, unspun)		
• White blood cells	0–4 WBC's/high power field	↑ in most UTIs
• Gram stain	None	↑ in most UTIs
STOOL EXAMINATION		
• Mucus (or white cells on smear)	None or minimal	↑ in invasive processes (e.g., shigella) rather than toxin reactions (e.g., Staphylococcal food poisoning)
• Blood	None	↑ in shigella
CSF		
• Glucose	40–80 mg % (at least 1/2 blood glucose level)	Usually low in bacterial meningitis
• Protein	5–40 mg % (up to 150 mg % in newborns)	Usually high in bacterial meningitis
• Cell count	0–7 lymphocytes (up to 25 in infants under 1 month)	↑ lymphocytes (e.g., TB, fungal, viral meningitis) ↑ polys (e.g., bacterial meningitis)
• Gram stain	No organisms	Bacterial organisms bacterial meningitis)
X RAYS, SCANS THERMOGRAPHY, ULTRASOUND	Normal anatomy	Abscesses or cyst (e.g., liver, lung) Infiltrates (e.g., pneumonia) Bony abnormalities (e.g., osteomyelitis)
THERAPEUTIC TRIAL		Clinical response may suggest correct diagnosis
SKIN TESTS	Test-specific and variable (*Note:* of little value in confirming ongoing infection)	↑ in many infections

SPECIFIC TESTS

Test	Normal Range	Abnormal Findings in Selected Diseases
CULTURES		
• **Urine**	$0-10^4$ bacteria/ml	$\geqslant 10^5$ organisms of single species
• **Blood, CSF, synovial fluid**	No growth	Pathogens
• **Sputum, stool, etc.**	Normal flora (see page 198)	Pathogens
GRAM STAINS IN CERTAIN SITUATIONS		
• **Male urethral discharge**	No organisms	Gram-negative, intracellular diplococci (e.g., gonorrhea)
SEROLOGY	Usually less than 1/8 but depends on test (*Note:* Some tests and titer changes allow confirmation.)	↑ in many infections (see page 207)

MANAGEMENT MODALITIES

Successful management of a patient with an infectious disease requires not only the selection of appropriate antimicrobial therapy when indicated, but also the use of a variety of management modalities that increase patient comfort, promote healing, and prevent spread to others at risk.

Therapeutic Objective	Clinical Problem	Therapy
Patient Comfort	Psychological stress	Patient education and emotional support
	Fever	Tepid water baths or sponging Antipyretics (e.g., aspirin, acetomenophin)
	Pain	Analgesics
	Swelling (e.g., of extremity)	Elevation and topical heat
	Sore throat	Gargles with salt water
	Ear ache (e.g., otitis externa)	Acidic solution (e.g., vinegar and water)
	(e.g., otitis media)	Hyperosmotic solution (e.g., warm sugar solution)
Promotion of Natural Healing Processes	Crusting	Wet compresses, debridement
	Poor blood supply	Moist controlled hot compresses
	Fatigue	Rest
	Dehydration	Rehydration (e.g., oral solution of: 1-1/2 qt water 1/4 tsp NaCl 1/2 cup sugar)
	Vaginal infection	Douching (e.g., vinegar and water solution)
Removal of Organisms and Foreign Bodies	Abscesses	Soaks, heat, I & D
	Foreign bodies	Removal of splinters, sutures, catheters, etc.
	Crusts	Soaks, compresses, debridement
Organism-Specific Therapy	Presence of pathogens	Antimicrobial therapy (see page 171)
Prevention of Spread to Others At Risk	Transmission of organisms	Isolation procedures (see page 232) Education on hygiene Human waste disposal Environmental control: water purification, proper food handling Immunizations (see page 218)

2

SELECTED DISEASE ENTITIES

▶ CLINICAL MANIFESTATIONS

1. Usually asymptomatic. Symptomatic intestinal invasion; rare below age 10; causes diarrhea (occasionally bloody); flatulence and crampy abdominal pain. Intermittent constipation common.
2. Hepatic abscess with right upper quadrant tenderness; fullness; occasional abrupt onset of high fevers (95% of abscesses are single and in right lobe of liver).

▶ EPIDEMIOLOGY

Agent: Parasitic—*Entamoeba histolytica,* a protozoa.

Reservoir: Humans.

Transmission: Usually by fecal-oral route, possibly contaminated food or water.

Incubation period: Unpredictable; usually 2–4 weeks.

Period of communicability: While cysts appear in the stools.

▶ DIAGNOSTIC PROCEDURES

Serology: Indirect hemagglutination tests are positive in all patients with hepatic abscesses and some with acute dysentery, but fail to distinguish between past and present infections.

Skin tests: Correlate well with serological tests, but are not useful clinically.

Other: Stool sample in saline should be examined immediately for mobile trophozoites. Methylene blue stain is helpful. As many as six specimens may be required. Antibiotics, antacids, enemas, and barium interfere with the recovery of the organisms. Sigmoidoscopy reveals ulcerations. Liver scan, ultrasound, or computerized axiotomography help detect hepatic abscesses (biopsy confirms diagnosis).*

▶ MANAGEMENT

Patient treatment

1. Intestinal carriers (asymptomatic)
   Diloxanide furoate 500 mg PO tid x 10 days
   (children: 20 mg/kg/day) *or*
   Metronidazole 750 mg PO tid x 5 days
   (children: 50 mg/kg/day).
2. Dysentery (intestinal infection) or abscesses (usually hepatic).
   Metronidazole alone cures 90% of cases.

(Continued on next page)

---

*Preserve specimens in 2 vials (PVA and formalin).

▶ MANAGEMENT (Cont.)

Addition of emetine hydrochloride (or dehydroemetine dihydrochloride) 60 mg/day IM x 10 days may be required in severe infections (children: 1 mg/kg/day).

Patient isolation: Enteric precautions (see page 233).

Management of contacts: Stool examinations for household members or others exposed to possible common source.

Other: Water can be treated with 5 drops tincture of iodine/qt (wait 30 minutes) to kill cysts. Avoid uncooked vegetables in endemic areas.

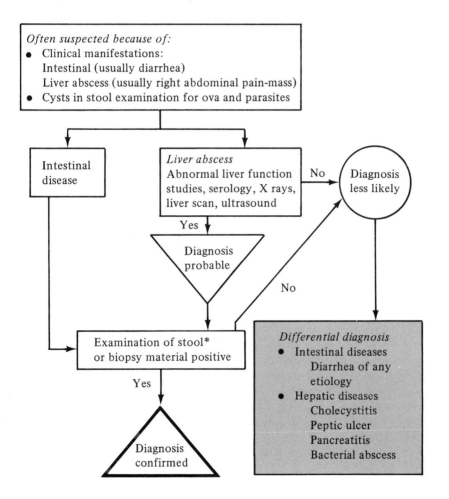

Often suspected because of:
- Clinical manifestations:
  Intestinal (usually diarrhea)
  Liver abscess (usually right abdominal pain-mass)
- Cysts in stool examination for ova and parasites

Intestinal disease

Liver abscess
Abnormal liver function studies, serology, X rays, liver scan, ultrasound

No → Diagnosis less likely

Yes ↓

Diagnosis probable

No

Examination of stool* or biopsy material positive

Yes ↓

Diagnosis confirmed

Differential diagnosis
- Intestinal diseases
  Diarrhea of any etiology
- Hepatic diseases
  Cholecystitis
  Peptic ulcer
  Pancreatitis
  Bacterial abscess

*Several daily stool examinations and sigmoid aspiration or biopsy may be required.

▶ **CLINICAL MANIFESTATIONS**

1. Usually asymptomatic
2. Massive infestation may cause abdominal pain, vomiting, malnutrition, and intestinal obstruction. The pulmonary phase of the worm's life cycle may cause pneumonitis with fever, cough, and migratory pulmonary infiltrates.

▶ **EPIDEMIOLOGY**

Agent: Parasitic—*Ascaris lumbricoides,* a helminth.

Reservoir: Humans.

Transmission: By ingestion of ascaris eggs in soil or contaminated food, after eggs have incubated several days.

Incubation period: 2 months.

Period of communicability: Until all fertile female worms are destroyed and stools are negative.

▶ **DIAGNOSTIC PROCEDURES**

Other: Ova and/or worms may be found in stools or vomitus. Blood eosinophilia common. Ascaris pneumonia may be diagnosed by observing larvae and eosinophilia in sputum.

▶ **MANAGEMENT**

Patient treatment: Piperazine citrate 7 mg/kg up to 4 gm each morning for 2 days, or pyrantel pamoate 11 mg/kg once daily x 3 days, or mebendazole 100 mg PO x 3 days.

Patient isolation: None. Not transmitted person to person.

Management of contacts: None, but other household members often infested.

Other: Encourage use of toilet facilities.

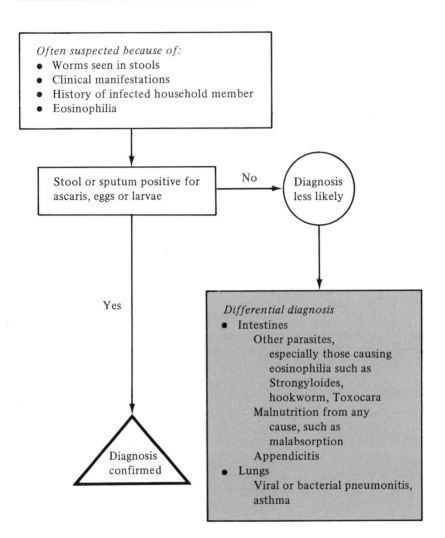

Often suspected because of:
- Worms seen in stools
- Clinical manifestations
- History of infected household member
- Eosinophilia

Stool or sputum positive for ascaris, eggs or larvae

No → Diagnosis less likely

Yes

Diagnosis confirmed

Differential diagnosis
- Intestines
    Other parasites, especially those causing eosinophilia such as Strongyloides, hookworm, Toxocara
    Malnutrition from any cause, such as malabsorption
    Appendicitis
- Lungs
    Viral or bacterial pneumonitis, asthma

► **CLINICAL MANIFESTATIONS**

1. Extremely variable. Often begins insidiously with fever, malaise, arthralgias, myalgias, headaches, weakness, sweating and chills, lasting a few weeks or months. A chronic stage may follow with weakness, aches, fever, and other psychoneurotic-like symptoms lasting for years. Relapses may occur.
2. Nonpurulent meningitis, pneumonitis, orchitis, and vertebral osteomyelitis may occur, but are uncommon.

Note: Clinical diagnosis is difficult.

► **EPIDEMIOLOGY**

Agent: Bacterial—species of the genus Brucella.

Reservoir: Most commonly cattle (*B. abortus*), hogs (*B. suis*), goats (*B. melitensis*), and laboratory dogs (*B. canis*).

Transmission: Usually by direct contact with infected animals and their blood, placentas, or urine (especially meat packers, farmworkers, veterinarians). Occasionally, ingestion of unpasteurized milk or cheese.

Incubation period: Extremely variable but usually 1–6 weeks.

Period of communicability: Not transmitted person to person.

Duration of immunity: Uncertain.

► **DIAGNOSTIC PROCEDURES**

Cultures: Specimens—Lymph nodes and bone marrow.
Media—Trypticase soy broth or tryptose phosphate broth.
Note: Cultures are often negative during chronic disease.

Serology: The card test is a useful agglutination screening test. Tube agglutination titers of 1 : 100 or more suggest active infection, but comparing acute and convalescent sera is best. (See page 207.)

Skin tests: Unreliable.

► **MANAGEMENT**

Patient treatment: Tetracycline, 500 mg PO qid for 3 weeks or more. For severe infections, also use streptomycin 500 mg bid.

Patient isolation: None.

Immunization: None for humans. Vaccine for cattle are of little value.

Other: Pasteurization of dairy products and elimination of infected animals is the major method of control. Protective procedures recommended for slaughterhouse workers, dairymen, veterinarians and other exposed individuals.

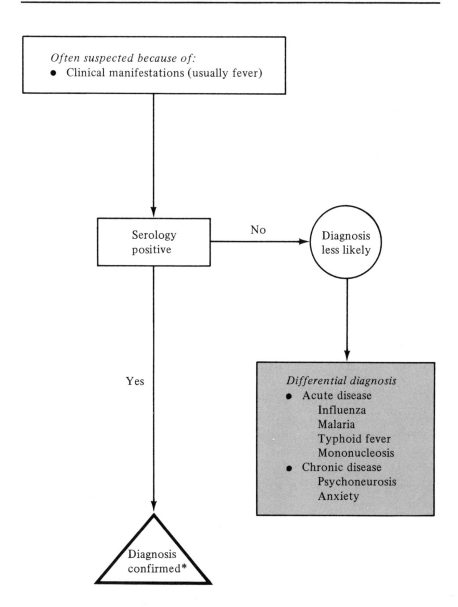

Often suspected because of:
- Clinical manifestations (usually fever)

Serology positive

No

Diagnosis less likely

Yes

Differential diagnosis
- Acute disease
  Influenza
  Malaria
  Typhoid fever
  Mononucleosis
- Chronic disease
  Psychoneurosis
  Anxiety

Diagnosis confirmed*

*False-positive serology caused by tularemia, cholera,
and rickettsial infections. Further confirmation
depends on cultures.

▶ **CLINICAL MANIFESTATIONS**

1. Skin: erythematous macular lesions with "satellites."
2. Oral: thrush, perleche.
3. Vaginal: thick, white discharge.
4. Balanitis.
5. Intestinal involvement commonly asymptomatic.
6. Lung: pneumonia.

▶ **EPIDEMIOLOGY**

Agent: Fungal, usually *Candida albicans.*

Reservoir: Primarily humans, but the fungus is ubiquitous.

Transmission: By self-inoculation, by direct person-to-person contact, and possibly by indirect contact with contaminated articles.

Incubation period: Variable.

Period of communicability: For duration of lesions.

▶ **DIAGNOSTIC PROCEDURES**

Cultures: Specimens.
         Media—Sabouraud's media.

Serology: Not clinically useful.

Skin tests: Not diagnostically useful.

Other: Microscopic demonstration of yeast cells or pseudohyphae by gram staining or contrast using a drop of ink or charcoal solution. Use 10% KOH to dissolve epithelial cells.

▶ **MANAGEMENT**

Patient treatment:

1. Oral or gastrointestinal disease—nystatin solution, 2–6 cc PO qid.
2. Skin disease—nystatin ointment or cream applied topically qid, aqueous gentian violet (1%) applied daily, or miconazole nitrate 2% cream.
3. Vaginal disease—nystatin vaginal suppositories, applied bid for 10 days.* White vinegar and water douche bid.
4. Systemic disease—amphotericin B (see page 167).

Patient isolation: None.

Management of contacts: None.

*Clotrimazole, 1 vaginal tablet qhs x 7 days.

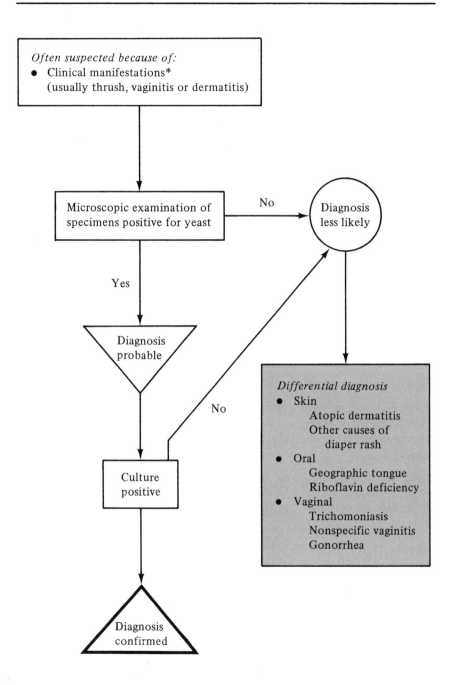

Often suspected because of:
- Clinical manifestations*
  (usually thrush, vaginitis or dermatitis)

Microscopic examination of specimens positive for yeast

No → Diagnosis less likely

Yes

Diagnosis probable

No

Culture positive

Differential diagnosis
- Skin
    Atopic dermatitis
    Other causes of
        diaper rash
- Oral
    Geographic tongue
    Riboflavin deficiency
- Vaginal
    Trichomoniasis
    Nonspecific vaginitis
    Gonorrhea

Diagnosis confirmed

*The clinical picture alone is often adequate to warrant therapy.

► CLINICAL MANIFESTATIONS

1. Infection may be asymptomatic, or may cause sudden onset of "rice water" stools. *No fever.*
2. Dehydration with acidosis and hypokalemia are common.

► EPIDEMIOLOGY

Agent: Bacterial—*Vibrio cholerae.* Inaba and Ogawa serotypes most common.

Reservoir: Humans.

Transmission: By ingestion of water (less commonly food) contaminated by feces, vomitus, patients, or carriers. Rarely spread directly person to person.

Incubation period: A few hours to 5 days.

Period of communicability: Until a few days after recovery. Several months for some carriers.

Duration of immunity: Poorly understood. Partial immunity may develop.

► DIAGNOSTIC PROCEDURES

Cultures: Specimens—feces and vomitus.
           Media—GTT or TCBS.
           Transport in Cary-Blair media.

Serology: Vibriocidal or agglutination titers are useful clinically.

Other: Darkfield or phase microscopy with vibrio immobilization antiserum may allow rapid identification.

► MANAGEMENT

Patient treatment: Oral fluid therapy with solution containing 3.5. gm NaCl, 2.5 gm $NaHCO_3$, 1.5 gm KCl, and 20 gm glucose/liter to make up rectal losses. IVs may be required. Tetracycline may be beneficial, but rarely indicated.

Patient isolation: Enteric precautions (see page 233).

Immunization: Gives short-lived (several months) protection, does not prevent asymptomatic infections, and has no useful role in disease control. May be required by some countries for international travel (see page 227).

Management of contacts: Do not immunize, but treat household contacts with tetracycline or furazolidone and observe 5 days for symptoms.

Other: Pure water supplies are the key to control (chlorination or boiling kills vibrios). All cases should be investigated for source.

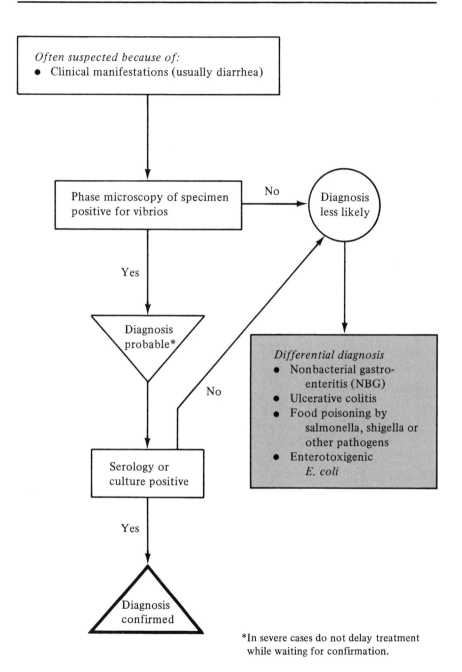

*In severe cases do not delay treatment
while waiting for confirmation.

▶ **CLINICAL MANIFESTATIONS**

1. Fever, lymphadenopathy, severe headache, and muscle, joint, and retro-orbital pain. Diffuse maculopapular rash is seen in less than 50% of cases.
2. Hemorrhagic fever with petechiae, epistaxis, and gastrointestinal and pulmonary hemorrhages. This complication is rare in the western hemisphere and is thought to be related to simultaneous infection by two types of dengue virus or to previous sensitization by one type followed by infection of another type.

▶ **EPIDEMIOLOGY**

Agent: Viral—one of four types of dengue virus, a group B arbovirus.

Reservoir: Humans and the *Aedes aegypti* mosquito.

Transmission: By the mosquitos which were infected by biting dengue fever patients at least 8–11 days previously.

Incubation period: Usually 5–6 days, but may be as long as 2 weeks.

Period of communicability: Not directly transmitted from person to person. Patients are infective for mosquitos from the day before onset to the fifth day of the disease.

Duration of immunity: Unknown, some type-specific immunity exists.

▶ **DIAGNOSTIC PROCEDURES**

Cultures: Specimen—blood and mosquitos.
          Media—animal inoculations.

Serology: Complement fixation titers are very useful clinically.

▶ **MANAGEMENT**

Patient treatment: Symptomatic.

Patient isolation: If practical, keep in screened rooms during first 5 days of illness.

Other: Mosquito surveillance control by use of screens, insecticides, and repellents; and elimination of breeding sites (such as garbage cans) in residential areas. Surveillance for additional cases in places of residency and travel during the week prior to onset of illness may help direct mosquito-control efforts.

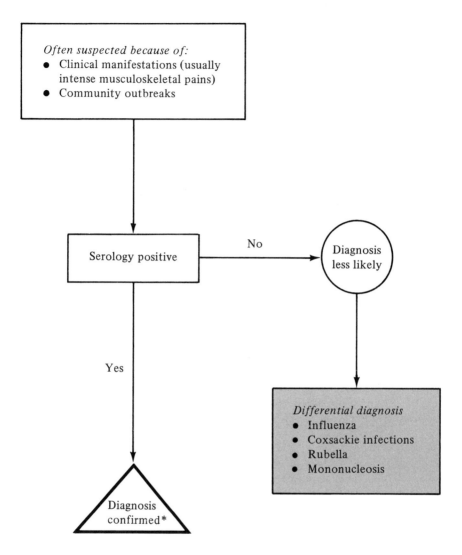

*Viral cultures can also confirm the diagnosis.

▶ CLINICAL MANIFESTATIONS

1. Superficial, spreading (often circular) skin lesions which are variably erythematous, vesicular and pustular, or papulosquamous.
2. Discolored and irregular nails.

▶ EPIDEMIOLOGY

Agent: Fungal—various microsporum, trichophyton, and epidermaphyton species.

Reservoir: Usually humans or domestic animals (for microsporum).

Transmission: Direct or indirect contact with infected people, animals, or contaminated articles.

Incubation period: Several days (e.g., Tinea corporis); 2 weeks (e.g., Tinea capitis); but often unknown (e.g., Tinea unguium).

Period of communicability: Duration of disease, extremely variable.

▶ DIAGNOSTIC PROCEDURES

Cultures: Specimens—skin scrapings, nails, hair.
            Media—Sabouraud's.

Other: Microscopic examination of scrapings in 10% potassium hydroxide (KOH) may show mycelia. Wood's light shows green fluorescence if agent is a microsporum.

▶ MANAGEMENT

Patient treatment:

1. Tinea capitis (scalp) and tinea barbae (beard)—griseofulvin (microcrystalline) 20 mg/kg/day (max. 1 gm daily) x 10 days.
2. Tinea unguium (nails)—griseofulvin for 6 months–2 years.
3. Tinea cruris (perineum) and tinea pedis (feet)
   Mild—Keep area dry, use loose cotton underwear, cotton socks and powder.
   Moderate—Include an undecylenic acid preparation (e.g., Cruex, Desenex) or a 30% aluminum chloride solution.
   Severe—Clotrimazole (e.g., Lotrimin) or miconazole (e.g., Micatin) topically. Rarely is griseofulvin required.
4. Tinea corporis (body other than above)—Tolnaftate (e.g., Tinactin), Whitfield's ointment (6% benzoic acid + 3% salicylic acid), or Selsun Blue shampoo used as cream.

Patient isolation: Not practical. Ideally, contact with infected persons or shared articles (clothes, towels) should be minimized.

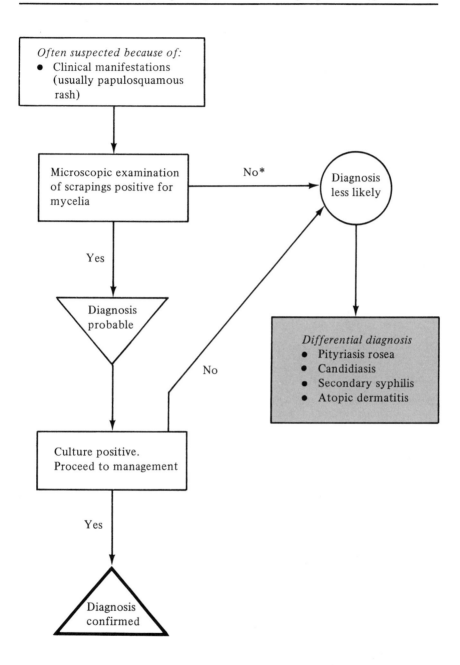

Often suspected because of:
- Clinical manifestations (usually papulosquamous rash)

Microscopic examination of scrapings positive for mycelia

No*

Diagnosis less likely

Yes

Diagnosis probable

No

Differential diagnosis
- Pityriasis rosea
- Candidiasis
- Secondary syphilis
- Atopic dermatitis

Culture positive. Proceed to management

Yes

Diagnosis confirmed

*Scrapings often negative in spite of infection.

▶ **CLINICAL MANIFESTATIONS**

1. Depends on site of infection:
   Pharynx—fever, sore throat, greyish "membrane," nuchal edema.
   Larynx—hoarseness, cough, respiratory obstruction.
   Nose—mucopurulent discharge.
   Skin—impetigo-like ulcers or abrasions.
2. The toxin may produce myocarditis, neuritis, paralysis, drowsiness, and delirium.

▶ **EPIDEMIOLOGY**

Agent: Bacterial—*Corynebacterium diphtheriae* and its toxins.

Reservoir: Humans.

Transmission: By direct contact with patient or carriers; indirect contact with contaminated articles such as clothes.

Incubation period: Usually 2–6 days, or longer.

Period of communicability: Less than 2 days in treated individuals, otherwise usually less than 2 weeks (6 months in some carriers).

Duration of immunity: Variable. Boosters recommended at least every 10 years.

▶ **DIAGNOSTIC PROCEDURES**

Cultures: Specimens—throat or skin lesion swab.
         Media—Loefflers, Tellurite, or blood agar plates.

Serology: Not clinically useful.

Skin tests: Schick test not clinically useful.

Other: Gram-staining specimens is not useful because of morphologic similarity to normal flora. Fluorescent antibody stains may allow rapid presumptive diagnosis.

▶ **MANAGEMENT**

Patient treatment: Penicillin or erythromycin. Antitoxin, 20,000–120,000 units IV, depending on severity of illness, is probably of little value for cutaneous diphtheria (test for hypersensitivity). Immunize cases with toxoid after recovery.

Patient isolation: Home restriction until two consecutive daily cultures are negative. Strict isolation for hospitalized patient (see page 232).

Immunization: Diphtheria toxoid as part of DPT at 2, 4, 6, 18 months, and 5 years; adult TD booster at least every 10 years.

Management of contacts

1. Examine and culture nose and throat of household and other close contacts. Check for skin lesions.

(Continued on next page)

► **MANAGEMENT (Cont.)**

2. Immunize contacts if not previously immunized or if last booster given more than 5 years earlier.
3. Treat intimate contacts with erythromycin for 7 days or with penicillin (IM or PO) if culture positive or unobtainable.
4. Home restriction of intimate contacts until cultures are proven negative.

Other: Hot water laundering of contaminated materials.

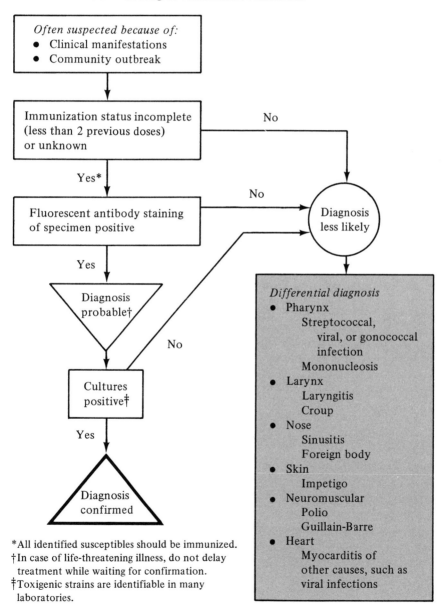

Often suspected because of:
• Clinical manifestations
• Community outbreak

Immunization status incomplete (less than 2 previous doses) or unknown

No

Yes*

Fluorescent antibody staining of specimen positive

No

Yes

Diagnosis less likely

Diagnosis probable†

No

Cultures positive‡

Yes

Diagnosis confirmed

Differential diagnosis
• Pharynx
   Streptococcal, viral, or gonococcal infection
   Mononucleosis
• Larynx
   Laryngitis
   Croup
• Nose
   Sinusitis
   Foreign body
• Skin
   Impetigo
• Neuromuscular
   Polio
   Guillain-Barre
• Heart
   Myocarditis of other causes, such as viral infections

*All identified susceptibles should be immunized.
†In case of life-threatening illness, do not delay treatment while waiting for confirmation.
‡Toxigenic strains are identifiable in many laboratories.

▶ **CLINICAL MANIFESTATIONS**

1. Often asymptomatic.
2. Perianal pruritus.
3. Scratching may cause perineal irritation, superinfection, and vulvovaginitis.
4. Salpingitis and abdominal pain may occur in females.

▶ **EPIDEMIOLOGY**

Agent: Parasitic—*Enterobius vermicularis,* an intestinal roundworm.

Reservoir: Humans.

Transmission: Fecal-oral route, primarily by hands, possibly by clothes and other articles or food.

Incubation period: Usually 2–6 weeks.

Period of communicability: As long as eggs are in the stool or perianal folds.

▶ **DIAGNOSTIC PROCEDURES**

Other: Cellophane tape applied briefly to the perianal region, removed, and observed microscopically may reveal eggs.

▶ **MANAGEMENT**

Patient treatment: Mebendazole (Vermox) 100 mg orally for children or adults, single dose. Alternatives include: pyrvinium pamoate (Povan), pyrantel (Antiminth), piperazine citrate, and thiabendazole. *Note:* If ascaris eggs are also present in the stool, treat with mebendazole 100 mg bid x 3 days (to prevent migration of adult worms). See Ascariasis.

Patient isolation: None.

Management of contacts: Consider simultaneous examination and/or treatment of household contacts, especially children, if reinfestation occurs.

Other: Special hygienic measures are frequently ineffective in preventing transmission. Laundering clothes and bedding at time of treatment may help prevent reinfestation.

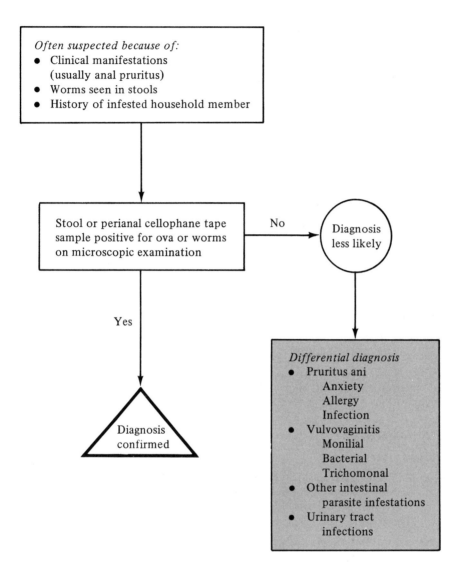

Often suspected because of:
- Clinical manifestations
  (usually anal pruritus)
- Worms seen in stools
- History of infested household member

Stool or perianal cellophane tape
sample positive for ova or worms
on microscopic examination

No → Diagnosis
less likely

Yes

Diagnosis
confirmed

Differential diagnosis
- Pruritus ani
    Anxiety
    Allergy
    Infection
- Vulvovaginitis
    Monilial
    Bacterial
    Trichomonal
- Other intestinal
    parasite infestations
- Urinary tract
    infections

► **CLINICAL MANIFESTATIONS**

Usually mild diarrhea with abdominal cramps. Occasionally nausea and vomiting, severe diarrhea, fever, malaise, and weight loss. Common cause of "travelers' diarrhea" and nursery epidemics.

► **EPIDEMIOLOGY**

Agent: Bacterial—*E. coli* (enteropathogenic serotypes and enterotoxigenic strains).

Reservoir: Humans.

Transmission: By fecal-oral route via contaminated hands or by consumption of contaminated food or water.

Incubation period: 2 hours–6 days.

Period of communicability: Variable, usually throughout period of infection. Individuals can become chronic carriers.

► **DIAGNOSTIC PROCEDURES**

Cultures: Specimens—stool.
Media—blood agar.

Note: Many laboratories cannot specifically identify toxin-producing strains of enteropathogenic serotypes. Tissue-culture tests are useful for outbreak investigations, but are not readily available.

► **MANAGEMENT**

Patient treatment

1. Infants—neomycin (100 mg/kg/day) or colistin (10–15 mg/kg/day) PO in 3 doses for at least 5 days and until culture negative.
2. Travelers—Supportive measures and fluid replacement (antibiotics usually not helpful).

Patient isolation: Keep infected individuals from children under 2 years. Enteric precautions for infected infants (see page 233).

Other: Handwashing and avoidance of consumption of contaminated water and inadequately cooked foods.

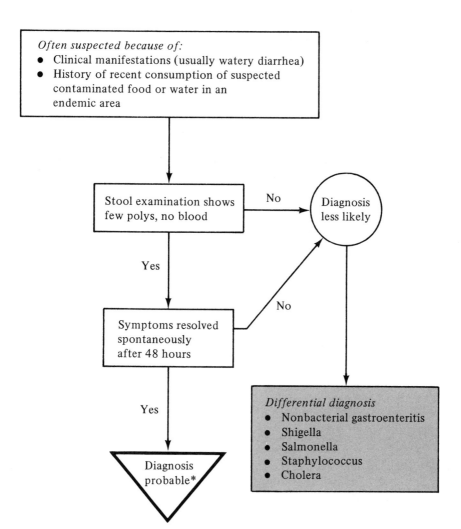

Often suspected because of:
- Clinical manifestations (usually watery diarrhea)
- History of recent consumption of suspected contaminated food or water in an endemic area

Stool examination shows few polys, no blood

No → Diagnosis less likely

Yes

Symptoms resolved spontaneously after 48 hours

No

Yes

Diagnosis probable*

Differential diagnosis
- Nonbacterial gastroenteritis
- Shigella
- Salmonella
- Staphylococcus
- Cholera

*If confirmation necessary for epidemiologic studies, perform tissue-culture tests for enterotoxin production.

▶ **CLINICAL MANIFESTATIONS**

Nausea, vomiting, diarrhea, abdominal pain, and fever. Outbreaks occur in all age groups, last for 1–2 days, and are often called "winter vomiting disease." Sporadic cases occur most commonly in those under age 4 and often lead to dehydration.

▶ **EPIDEMIOLOGY**

Agent: Viral—like the Norwalk and Hawaii agents (responsible for outbreaks of viral gastroenteritis) and the reovirus-like agents (responsible for sporadic cases).

Reservoir: Humans.

Transmission: Probably by fecal-oral route, direct contact between people, or by contaminated food and water.

Incubation period: 1–3 days.

Period of communicability: During acute illness, possibly for 2 weeks.

Duration of immunity: Unknown, probably agent-specific. Reinfection may occur.

▶ **DIAGNOSTIC PROCEDURES**

Cultures: None.

Serology: Immune electronmicroscopy complement fixation and/or immune fluorescent techniques available in some laboratories if absolute identification is required (outbreak investigation).

Other: Electronmicroscopy of stool, food, or water may help in investigations. Methylene blue stain of stools may show either no white blood cells or some monos.

▶ **MANAGEMENT**

Patient treatment: Symptomatic.

Patient isolation: Enteric precautions while ill (see page 233). Keep away from young children.

Other: Search for common sources.

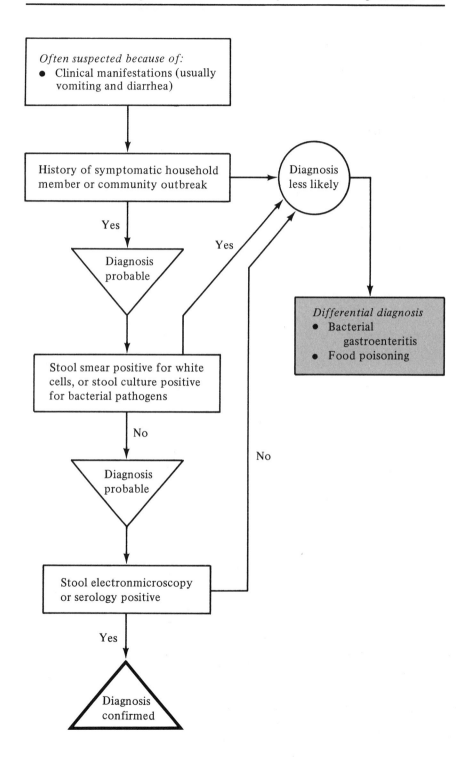

▶ **CLINICAL MANIFESTATIONS**

1. Often asymptomatic. Foul smelling, bulky stools, diarrhea, epigastric pain, flatulence, and nausea.
2. Weight loss and malabsorption may develop.

▶ **EPIDEMIOLOGY**

Agent: Parasitic—*Giardia lamblia,* a protozoa.

Reservoir: Humans, beavers.

Transmission: Fecal-oral route by contaminated hands, ingestion of contaminated water, and possibly food.

Incubation period: Variable, usually 1–3 weeks.

Period of communicability: Until cysts or trophozoites are no longer present in stools.

▶ **DIAGNOSTIC PROCEDURES**

Other: Direct examination of stool (multiple samples), duodenal washings, or jejunal biopsies for motile trophozoites on unstained, saline wet-mount. Preserve specimens in two vials (PVA and formalin).

▶ **MANAGEMENT**

Patient treatment: Quinacrine hydrochloride (Atabrine) 2 mg/kg/dose (100 mg max.) tid x 5 days, or metronidazole (Flagyl) 5 mg/kg/dose (250 mg max.) tid x 10 days.

Patient isolation: None.

Management of contacts: Evaluate stool specimens of household members.

Other: Attempt to find common water source for clusters of cases.

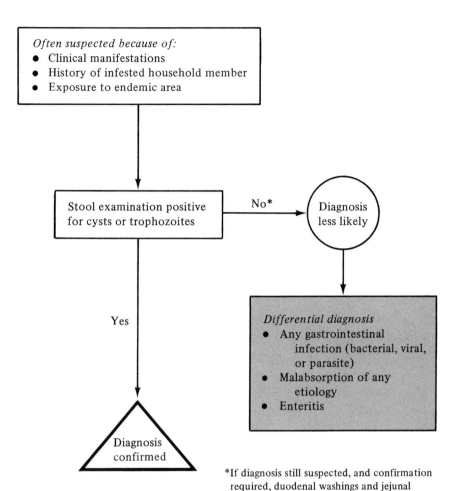

Often suspected because of:
- Clinical manifestations
- History of infested household member
- Exposure to endemic area

Stool examination positive for cysts or trophozoites

No*

Diagnosis less likely

Yes

Differential diagnosis
- Any gastrointestinal infection (bacterial, viral, or parasite)
- Malabsorption of any etiology
- Enteritis

Diagnosis confirmed

*If diagnosis still suspected, and confirmation required, duodenal washings and jejunal biopsies may be indicated.

▶ CLINICAL MANIFESTATIONS

1. Primary infections often asymptomatic. Clinical picture variable.
2. Males—Dysuria, urinary frequency, and purulent urethral discharge. Prostatitis and epididymitis may develop; proctitis in male homosexuals.
3. Females—Vaginal discharge and urinary frequency. Pelvic inflammatory disease (PID) and perihepatitis may develop with fever, abdominal pain, cramps, and vomiting.
4. Males and females—Pharyngitis is common.
5. Septicemia may lead to arthritis, meningitis, endocarditis, and/or dermatitis (papular, petechial, pustular, or necrotic skin lesions). Newborns of an infected mother may develop conjunctivitis.

▶ EPIDEMIOLOGY

Agent: Bacterial—*Neisseria gonorrhoeae.*

Reservoir: Humans.

Transmission: Sexual transmission to mucosal surfaces.

Incubation period: 3–5 days.

Period of communicability: For duration of presence of organisms.

▶ DIAGNOSTIC PROCEDURES

Cultures: Specimens—swabs from urethra, cervix, rectum, throat, and other sites as indicated.
Media—Thayer-Martin or Transgrow, promptly at room temperature, in CO_2.

Other: Gram stain of urethral discharge in males and conjunctival discharge in newborns are reliable, but cervical gram stains are unreliable.

▶ MANAGEMENT

Patient treatment

1. Uncomplicated, adult male or female.
   Procaine penicillin, 4.8 million units IM (two sites) plus probenicid 1 gm PO. Alternatives are: spectinomycin 2 gm IM; ampicillin 3.5 gm PO plus probenicid 1 gm PO; tetracycline 1.5 gm PO followed by 0.5 gm PO qid x 4 days, or erythromycin 1.5 gm PO followed by 0.5 gm PO qid x 4 days.
2. Uncomplicated, prepubertal female or male. Same as above but probenicid 25 mg/kg, procaine penicillin 100,000 units/kg, ampicillin 50 mg/kg, spectinomycin 40 mg/kg, tetracycline or erythromycin 25 mg/kg initial dose followed by 10 mg/kg/dose.
3. Pelvic inflammatory disease, mild—outpatient. Aqueous procaine penicillin G, 4.8 million units IM, or ampicillin 0.5 gm PO qid x 10 days.
4. Pelvic inflammatory disease, severe or disseminated infections. Aqueous crystalline penicillin G, IV 20 million units/day until clinical improvement followed by ampicillin 0.5 gm PO qid to complete 10 days' treatment. For penicillin-allergic patients, tetracycline 2.0 gm PO, daily x 10 days (IV in severe disease).

(Continued on next page)

▶ MANAGEMENT (Cont.)

5. Ophthalmia neonatorum (conjunctivitis in newborn). Aqueous crystalline penicillin G, IV 50,000 units/kg/day in 3 doses for 7 days, *plus* saline irrigations and instillation of penicillin, tetracycline, or chloramphenicol eyedrops.
6. Pharyngeal infection. Penicillin or tetracycline.

Patient isolation: None

Management of contacts: Identify, examine, culture, and treat all sexual partners of affected individuals. Males should refrain from intercourse or use condoms until 4 days after the onset of therapy.

Other: 1% silver nitrate eyedrops for all newborn infants helps prevent disease.

Often suspected because of:

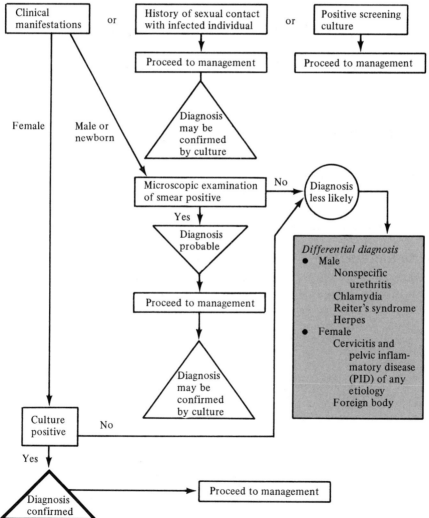

▶ **CLINICAL MANIFESTATIONS**

1. Slowly developing hypo- or hyperpigmented macules, papules, plaques, or nodules, often associated with anesthesias or paresthesias. Loss of temperature sensation is often an early manifestation.
   a. Lepromatous form—lesions are characterized as diffuse, most often occurring in the face, ears, wrist.
   b. Tuberculoid form—lesions more discrete, finely demarcated, associated with early nerve involvement.
   c. Borderline or intermediate form—variable lesions.

▶ **EPIDEMIOLOGY**

Agent: Bacterial—*Mycobacterium leprae,* an acid-fast bacteria.

Reservoir: Humans.

Transmission: Probably by direct, long-term, skin or mucus membrane contact with infected people.

Incubation period: 3 months–20 years. Usually several years.

Period of communicability: Unknown. The tuberculoid form is the least communicable.

▶ **DIAGNOSTIC PROCEDURES**

Serology: None. Patients may have false-positive serology for syphilis.

Skin tests: Lepromin (Mitsuda) test is never positive in lepromatous, but often positive in tuberculoid leprosy. Many false negatives.

Other: Smear, or biopsy of lesion may demonstrate acid-fast bacillus, granulomatous reactions, and large foam (Virchow's) cells.

▶ **MANAGEMENT**

Patient treatment: Traditionally treated with dapsone or DDS (4-diaminodiphenylsulfone) usually about 1 mg/kg/day up to 50 mg/day in adults. Treat lepromatous leprosy at least 10 years and tuberculoid disease at least 1–1-1/2 years. Rifampin may also be effective. Steroids and surgery are occasionally indicated. *Consult a leprologist.*

*Patient isolation:** Until the organism cannot be identified in lesions.

*Management of contacts:** Observation of household and other close contacts for manifestations.

Other: Education of public, stressing treatment availability and effectiveness.

*Consult the health department for specifics.

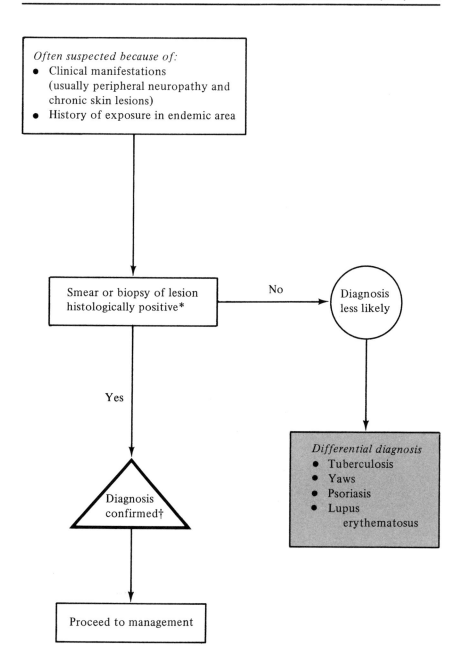

Often suspected because of:
- Clinical manifestations
  (usually peripheral neuropathy and
  chronic skin lesions)
- History of exposure in endemic area

Smear or biopsy of lesion
histologically positive*

No

Diagnosis
less likely

Yes

Diagnosis
confirmed†

Differential diagnosis
- Tuberculosis
- Yaws
- Psoriasis
- Lupus
  erythematosus

Proceed to management

*Should be performed by experienced physician.
†Culture or animal inoculation tests usually not available.

▶ **CLINICAL MANIFESTATIONS**

1. Commonly epiglottitis, pneumonia, otitis media, meningitis, conjunctivitis, sinusitis, facial (including periorbital) cellulitis.
2. Most common in children under 6 years of age.

▶ **EPIDEMIOLOGY**

Agent: Bacterial—*Hemophilus influenzae,* serotypes a–f (b and untypable are most common).

Reservoir: Humans.

Transmission: By direct contact, droplet spread, or indirectly by contaminated articles.

Incubation period: Not well-determined, probably several days.

Period of communicability: Duration of presence of organisim.

Duration of immunity: Unknown.

▶ **DIAGNOSTIC PROCEDURES**

Cultures: Specimens—depends on site affected.
            Media—chocolate agar in CO_2 atmosphere.

Serology: Not clinically useful.

Other: Gram staining useful (gram-negative pleomorphic rods). CIE of CSF may be useful in cases of meningitis.

▶ **MANAGEMENT**

Patient treatment: Ampicillin. Chloramphenicol for ampicillin-resistant strains or for severe infections if sensitivity unknown.

Patient isolation: Not necessary.

Immunization: Vaccine under development.

Management of contacts: None.

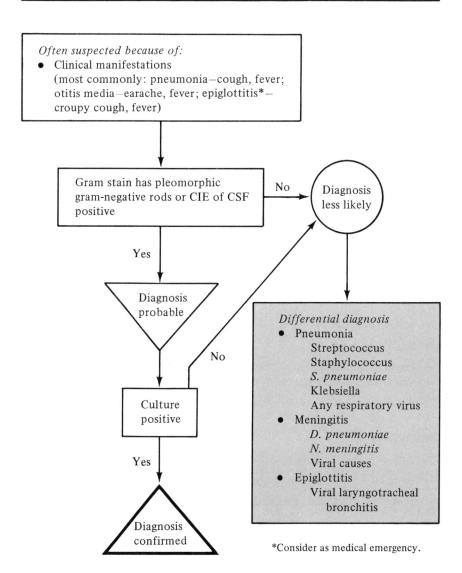

Often suspected because of:
- Clinical manifestations
  (most commonly: pneumonia—cough, fever;
  otitis media—earache, fever; epiglottitis*—
  croupy cough, fever)

Gram stain has pleomorphic gram-negative rods or CIE of CSF positive

No → Diagnosis less likely

Yes

Diagnosis probable

No

Culture positive

Yes

Diagnosis confirmed

Differential diagnosis
- Pneumonia
  Streptococcus
  Staphylococcus
  S. pneumoniae
  Klebsiella
  Any respiratory virus
- Meningitis
  D. pneumoniae
  N. meningitis
  Viral causes
- Epiglottitis
  Viral laryngotracheal
  bronchitis

*Consider as medical emergency.

▶ **CLINICAL MANIFESTATIONS**

1. Fever, abdominal pain, anorexia, and malaise. May be followed in several days by jaundice.
2. Mild, anicteric cases are common, especially in children.

▶ **EPIDEMIOLOGY**

Agent: Viral—hepatitis A virus.

Reservoir: Humans, occasionally other primates.

Transmission: Usually by fecal-oral route, or contact with feces, blood, urine, of infected individuals. Contaminated water or foods may cause common source outbreaks (especially milk, meats, shellfish).

Incubation period: From 2–7 weeks (usually about 4).

Period of communicability: Usually from 2 weeks before until 1–2 weeks after onset of jaundice.

Duration of immunity: Lifelong, hepatitis A type-specific.

▶ **DIAGNOSTIC PROCEDURES**

Cultures: None.

Serology: Radioimmune assay available in some laboratories. Serologic tests for hepatitis B antigen (HB Ag) only diagnostic of hepatitis B).

Other: Bilirubin, SGOT, SGPT (nonspecific tests that may be helpful).

▶ **MANAGEMENT**

Patient treatment: Supportive.

Patient isolation: Enteric precautions (see page 233).

Immunization: No active immunization available.

Management of contacts: Passive immunization with ISG (immune serum globulin) for:
1. Post-exposure household, institutional and other close contacts (dose 0.02 ml/kg IM). *Note:* School, hospital, office, or factory exposure usually is not significant.
2. Pre-exposure travelers to highly endemic areas (dose 0.05 ml/kg IM x 6 months).

Other measures: Environmental sanitation.

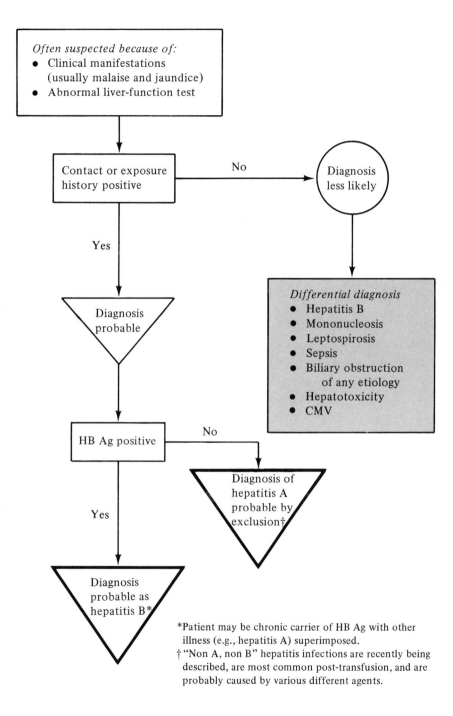

Often suspected because of:
- Clinical manifestations (usually malaise and jaundice)
- Abnormal liver-function test

Contact or exposure history positive

No → Diagnosis less likely

Yes

Diagnosis probable

Differential diagnosis
- **Hepatitis B**
- **Mononucleosis**
- **Leptospirosis**
- **Sepsis**
- **Biliary obstruction of any etiology**
- **Hepatotoxicity**
- **CMV**

HB Ag positive

No → Diagnosis of hepatitis A probable by exclusion†

Yes

Diagnosis probable as hepatitis B*

*Patient may be chronic carrier of HB Ag with other illness (e.g., hepatitis A) superimposed.

† "Non A, non B" hepatitis infections are recently being described, are most common post-transfusion, and are probably caused by various different agents.

▶ CLINICAL MANIFESTATIONS

Usually slow onset of malaise, abdominal pain, anorexia, nausea, vomiting, and jaundice, lasting up to 3 months.

▶ EPIDEMIOLOGY

Agent: Viral—hepatitis B virus.

Reservoir: Humans.

Transmission: Usually by transfusion or accidental inoculation or ingestion of contaminated blood products. Contaminated equipment (e.g., needles, dental instruments) are common sources of infection. Sexual or fecal-oral transmission may occur.

Incubation period: 6 weeks to 6 months.

Period of communicability: Usually several months, or as long as virus present in blood (occasionally years in chronic carriers).

Duration of immunity: May be lifelong, hepatitis B type-specific.

▶ DIAGNOSTIC PROCEDURES

Cultures: None.

Serology: Hepatitis B antigen (HB Ag) test usually positive. Antibodies to hepatitis B surface may appear later and demonstrate prior infection.

Other: Bilirubin, SGOT, SGPT, prothrombin time (none specific but helpful).

▶ MANAGEMENT

Patient treatment: Supportive.

Patient isolation: Enteric precautions only for hospitalized patients.

Immunization: No active immunization available.

Management of contacts

1. Use hepatitis B immune globulin (HBIG) when available, in place of serum globulin (ISG); use is controversial.
2. Postexposure prophylaxis with HBIG, 0.05–0.07 ml/kg IM within 7 days of exposure and repeat in 1 month, or ISG (same dose) for those with parenteral or mucosal exposure to known HB Ag positive blood.
3. Postexposure prophylaxis of infants born to mothers with acute hepatitis B in the third trimester and HB Ag seropositivity at time of delivery, HBIG 0.13 ml/kg IM single dose or ISG 0.5 ml/kg IM, within 7 days of exposure. Clean maternal blood from skin.

Other measures: Instruct those at risk of acquiring hepatitis B (e.g., hemo-dialysis and laboratory technicians, drug addicts) and those at risk of trans-mitting hepatitis B (e.g., dentists, blood donors) in appropriate control measures (e.g., use of gloves).

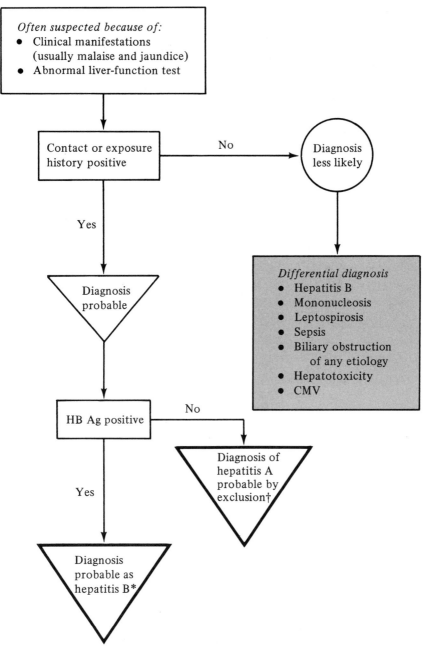

*Patient may be chronic carrier of HB Ag with other illness (e.g., hepatitis A) superimposed.

† "Non A, nonB" hepatitis infections are recently being described, are most common post-transfusion, and are probably caused by various different agents.

▶ CLINICAL MANIFESTATIONS

1. Primary infection is often subclinical, but may result in fever, malaise, gingivostomatitis, pharyngitis, keratoconjunctivitis, vulvovaginitis, and vesicular skin lesions. A meningoencephalitis with lateralizing signs mimicking a mass lesion may occur.
2. After a variable latent period, recurrent infections may be precipitated by various stimuli ranging from physical trauma to bacterial infections. Herpes labialis (cold sores), with blisters on the face and lips, and genital herpes are the most common recurrent forms.

▶ EPIDEMIOLOGY

Agent: Viral—herpes simplex virus (HSV) type 1 for most nongenital infections. HSV type 2 for most genital lesions.

Reservoir: Humans.

Transmission: By direct contact, especially sexual contact for type 2.

Incubation period: From 2 days to 2 weeks.

Period of communicability: While lesions are present, possibly several weeks. Asymptomatic persons may shed virus intermittently.

Duration of immunity: None of clinical significance.

▶ DIAGNOSTIC PROCEDURES

Cultures: Specimens—swabs of lesions, saliva, urine, genital secretions; brain biopsy (encephalitis).
Media—tissue culture.

Serology: Neutralizing antibody titers may be clinically useful and differentiate between type 1 and type 2 infections.

Skin tests: None.

Other: Scraping (including Pap smears) may reveal intranuclear inclusions or giant cells. Electronmicroscopy may reveal virus particles.

▶ MANAGEMENT

Patient treatment

1. Labial lesions—none.
2. Genital lesions—none except for sitbaths and drying.
3. Corneal lesions—5 IDU.
4. Disseminated infections and encephalitis—adenine arabinoside IV may be beneficial.

(Continued on next page)

▶ MANAGEMENT (Cont.)

Patient isolation: Keep infected persons away from newborns, those with severe eczema or burns, and immunodeficient or suppressed patients. If in hospital, respiratory isolation for oral disease (see page 232).

Immunization: None.

Other

1. Education about limiting indiscriminate sexual relations may help prevent genital herpes.
2. Cesarean section, for women with primary or recurrent disease at time of delivery, to prevent neonatal herpes.

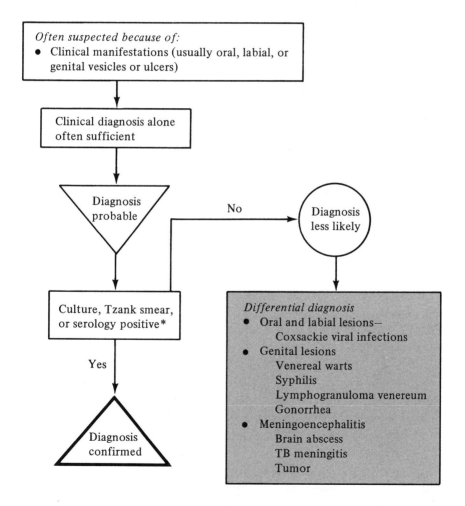

Often suspected because of:
- Clinical manifestations (usually oral, labial, or genital vesicles or ulcers)

Clinical diagnosis alone often sufficient

Diagnosis probable

No → Diagnosis less likely

Culture, Tzank smear, or serology positive*

Yes

Diagnosis confirmed

Differential diagnosis
- Oral and labial lesions—
   Coxsackie viral infections
- Genital lesions
   Venereal warts
   Syphilis
   Lymphogranuloma venereum
   Gonorrhea
- Meningoencephalitis
   Brain abscess
   TB meningitis
   Tumor

*Serology may be useful in initial infection, but not in recurrent disease.

▶ CLINICAL MANIFESTATIONS

1. Initial infection is usually asymptomatic.
2. Acute, mild, self-limited respiratory disease with some fever, malaise, and cough.
3. Acute disseminated disease with fever, prostration, hepatosplenomegaly, and erythema nodosum.
4. Chronic disseminated disease with varying symptoms of fever, pneumonia, hepatitis, endocarditis, and meningitis.
5. Chronic pulmonary disease resembling chronic pulmonary tuberculosis.

▶ EPIDEMIOLOGY

Agent: Fungal—*Histoplasma capsulatum.*

Reservoir: Soil and dust contaminated by droppings of bats and birds such as chickens and starlings. Caves and chickenhouses are common sources.

Transmission: By inhalation of airborne spores.

Incubation period: 5–18 days.

Period of communicability: Not usually transmitted from person to person.

Duration of immunity: Previous exposure may afford some resistance to infection.

▶ DIAGNOSTIC PROCEDURES

Cultures: Specimens—blood, sputum, urine, bone marrow, and other sites.
Biopsies and bronchial washings or brushings may be useful.
Media—Sabouraud's media at room temperature.

Serology: Complement fixation (histoplasmin skin tests and various fungal infections may cause false-positive results).

Skin tests: Histoplasmin test useful only for screening groups and may affect serology.

Other: Microscopic examination of specimens stained with Giemsa, Wright's, or acid Schiff stain. Chest X ray—variable, usually infiltrates, may also be miliary, coin, or cavitary lesions.

▶ MANAGEMENT

Patient treatment: Asymptomatic or mild infection—no treatment. Disseminated or chronic infections—amphotericin B (see page 167) for dosage and administration protocol).

Patient isolation: None.

Other: Avoid bat-infested caves and minimize time spent in enclosed contaminated areas such as chickenhouses. Spraying dust or dirt with water may reduce transmission. 3% formalin solution kills the fungus. Cases should be investigated to determine the source of infection.

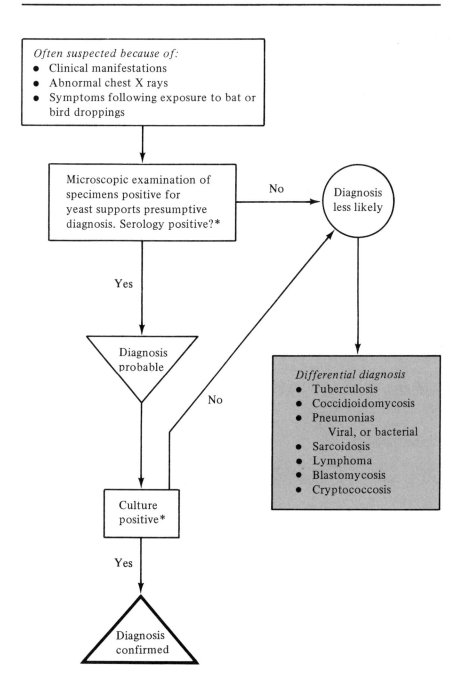

Often suspected because of:
- Clinical manifestations
- Abnormal chest X rays
- Symptoms following exposure to bat or bird droppings

Microscopic examination of specimens positive for yeast supports presumptive diagnosis. Serology positive?*

No → Diagnosis less likely

Yes

Diagnosis probable

No

Culture positive*

Yes

Diagnosis confirmed

Differential diagnosis
- Tuberculosis
- Coccidioidomycosis
- Pneumonias
  Viral, or bacterial
- Sarcoidosis
- Lymphoma
- Blastomycosis
- Cryptococcosis

*Do not delay treatment in severe, life-threatening infections while awaiting laboratory results.

▶ CLINICAL MANIFESTATIONS

1. Usually asymptomatic, but may cause chronic malnutrition, anemia, growth and developmental retardation, and various GI symptoms.
2. Migrating larvae cause dermatitis (especially of feet), cough, and wheezing.

▶ EPIDEMIOLOGY

Agent: Parasitic—*Necator americanus* and *Ancylostoma duodenale.*

Reservoir: Humans.

Transmission:

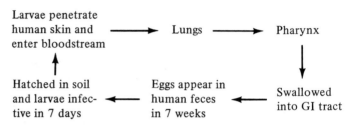

Incubation period: Weeks to months.

Period of communicability: As long as eggs are in stool (may be years) and larvae are in soil (may be weeks).

▶ DIAGNOSTIC PROCEDURES

Other: Identification of adult worms, larvae, or ova in stools.

▶ MANAGEMENT

Patient treatment: Pyrantel pamoate 11 mg/kg PO (max. 1 gm) once a day for 3 days. Alternatives include bephenium, tetrachloroethylene, or thiabendazole.

Patient isolation: None.

Management of contacts: None, but other household members are often infested.

Other measures: Sanitary disposal of human feces. Wearing of shoes.

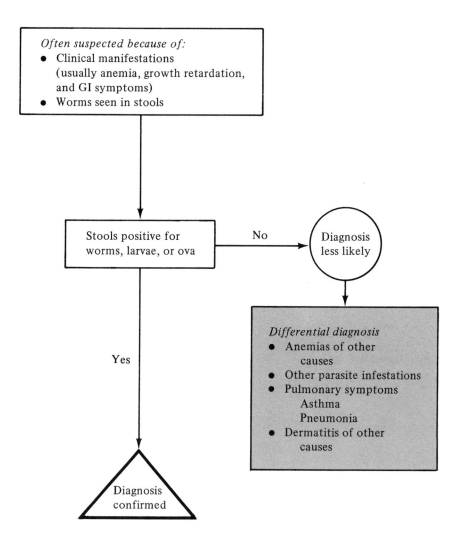

▶ **CLINICAL MANIFESTATIONS**

1. Fever, chills, myalgias, cough, coryza, and sore throat.
2. Severe disease and bacterial superinfection may occur, especially in those at high risk (see below, Immunization).

▶ **EPIDEMIOLOGY**

Agent: Viral—the influenza virus, usually types A and B, with numerous antigenically distinct strains.

Reservoir: Primarily humans. Other mammals serve as reservoir for new strains. strains.

Transmission: By direct contact, droplet spread, airborne, and articles contaminated by respiratory secretions.

Incubation period: From a day or so before, to 1 week after onset of symptoms.

Duration of immunity: Variable. Immunity is strain-specific but does offer some protection against related strains.

▶ **DIAGNOSTIC PROCEDURES**

Cultures: Specimens—washings from oropharynx.
　　　　　 Media—tissue cultures.

Serology: CF, HI, and neutralization techniques are useful. Compare acute and convalescent (2 weeks later) sera.

Skin tests: None.

Other: Immunofluorescent staining of nasal smears is possible.

▶ **MANAGEMENT**

Patient treatment: Nonspecific, symptomatic. Treat bacterial superinfections.

Patient isolation: None. Keep high-risk individuals away from those suspected of having influenza.

Immunization: An inactivated virus vaccine, with strains antigenically similar to those expected to produce epidemics in the coming "season," is recommended *yearly* for those at high risk: (1) the elderly—over 60; (2) those with chronic heart disease, including rheumatic, severe congenital, hypertensive; (3) those with chronic lung disease, including asthma, cystic fibrosis, emphysema; (4) those with chronic renal, neurologic, and metabolic disorders (including diabetes; (5) those with malignancies and immunodeficiencies; (6) institutionalized children.

Vaccine may cause malaise and fever. Febrile seizures may occur in children under 3. Two doses of "split product" vaccines (4 weeks apart) recommended for children under 12.

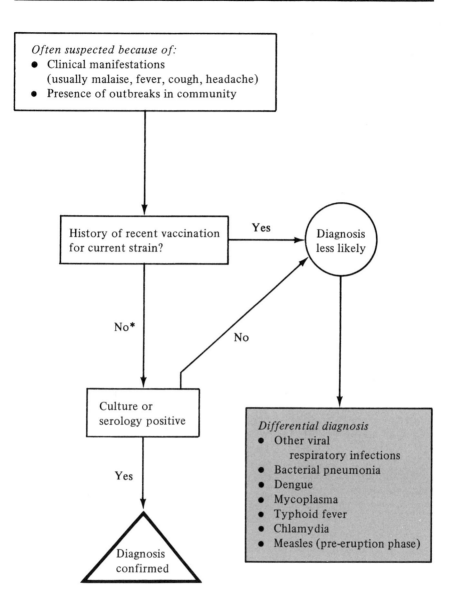

*Vaccinate if in high-risk group and early in "season."

▶ **CLINICAL MANIFESTATIONS**

1. Often asymptomatic. Extremely variable, with headache, vomiting, muscle cramps, jaundice, conjunctivitis, and fever.
2. Petechial rash, meningitis, hemolytic anemia, and renal failure may occur.

▶ **EPIDEMIOLOGY**

Agent: Bacterial—Leptospira serotypes (*L. icterohaemorrhagiae, L. canicola,* or *L. pomona*).

Reservoir: Domestic and wild animals.

Transmission: By broken skin or mucus membrane contact with urine of infected animals or with contaminated materials, including water.

Incubation period: 2–20 days, usually 10 days.

Period of communicability: Usually not transmitted from person to person.

▶ **DIAGNOSTIC PROCEDURES**

Cultures: Specimens—blood during acute illness, urine after first week.
Media—Fletcher's, bovine albumin polysorbate, animal inoculation.

Serology: Macroscopic slide agglutination (easy but not sensitive). Agglutination and complement fixation titer increases can confirm the diagnosis.

▶ **MANAGEMENT**

Patient treatment: Penicillin, erythromycin, or tetracycline may be of benefit if started during first few days of illness.

Patient isolation: None

Other: Determine source of infection (e.g., farm pond). Warn against swimming in contaminated waters.

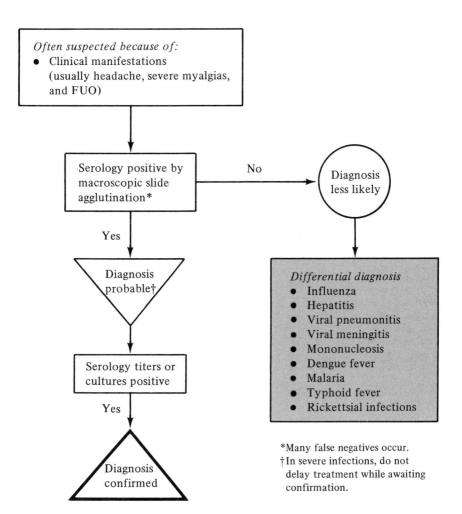

Often suspected because of:
- Clinical manifestations
  (usually headache, severe myalgias,
  and FUO)

Serology positive by macroscopic slide agglutination*

No → Diagnosis less likely

Yes

Diagnosis probable†

Serology titers or cultures positive

Yes

Diagnosis confirmed

Differential diagnosis
- Influenza
- Hepatitis
- Viral pneumonitis
- Viral meningitis
- Mononucleosis
- Dengue fever
- Malaria
- Typhoid fever
- Rickettsial infections

*Many false negatives occur.
†In severe infections, do not
  delay treatment while awaiting
  confirmation.

▶ **CLINICAL MANIFESTATIONS**

Classically with fever, shaking, chills, sweating, and headache often occurring in cycles every 1, 2, or 3 days. Vague flu-like symptoms are common. Recurrences may occur.

▶ **EPIDEMIOLOGY**

Agent: Parasitic—the four blood parasites: *Plasmodium vivax* (P.v.), *P. malariae* (P.m.), *P. falciparum* (P.f.), and *P. ovale* (P.o., Africa only).

Reservoir: Humans.

Transmission: By the bite of an infected mosquito (Anopheles spp.), transfusion of blood products from infected people, and use of contaminated needles.

Incubation period: About 12–14 days for P.f., P.v., and P.o., and 30 days for P.m. Shorter in cases caused by transfusions.

Period of communicability: Within 3–14 days after onset of symptoms, the blood of man is infectious for mosquitos (which remain infected for life—about 1 month). If not completely treated, patients may remain infectious for 1 year with P.f., for 3 years with P.v., and for life with P.m.

Duration of immunity: None, but some people exposed over a long time may develop some tolerance or resistance.

▶ **DIAGNOSTIC PROCEDURES**

Serology: Fourfold rise in FA titers may help, but acute specimens are rarely available.

Other: Microscopic examination of both thick and thin film blood smears for parasites.

▶ **MANAGEMENT**

Patient treatment

1. For P.v., P.m., P.o. and "chloroquine sensitive" P.f., chloroquine phosphate orally 1 gm (contains 600 mg of base), then 500 mg in 6 hours, and then 500 mg daily for 2–5 days.
2. For malaria of unknown type or for "chloroquine resistant" P.f., quinine sulfate, 650 mg PO q8h x 10 days, or quinine dihydrochloride 600 mg IV (if PO not tolerated) diluted in a liter of normal saline given over several hours for no more than three of the doses, then followed by PO meds. (Infants under 1 year, give 10% adult dose.
Children 1–15 years old, use age/20 x adult dose)
plus
pyrimethamine 25 mg PO q12h for 3 days (children under 1 year, 3 mg; 1–3 years, 6 mg; 4–6 years, 9 mg; 7–11 years, 12 mg)
plus
sulfadiazine 2.0 gm PO initially; then 500 mg q6h for 5 days (children, 100–150 mg/kg/day).

(Continued on next page)

▶ MANAGEMENT (Cont.)

Patient isolation: None. Keep patients away from mosquitos by screening or spraying if possible.

Management of contacts

1. Observe mosquito-exposed household members for symptoms.
2. Prophylaxis for most travelers: chloroquine phosphate 500 mg PO once weekly (children: 5 mg base/kg/week). Crush and dissolve 500 mg tablet in 40 cc chocolate syrup (each tsp will contain 37.5 mg base). Start 1 week prior to and continue for 8 weeks after exposure. Most attacks occur within 1 year of exposure.
3. If intense exposure has occurred, consider primaquine phosphate, 26.3 mg (15 mg base)/day PO x 14 days (children: 0.3 mg base/kg/day).
4. Prophylaxis for travelers to Panama, northern South America and SE Asia where chloroquine-resistant P.f. occurs: use pyrimethamine 25 mg plus sulfadoxine 500 mg, PO once a week (available in combination as Fansidar outside of US).

Other: Mosquito surveillance and eradication. Screening of blood donors.

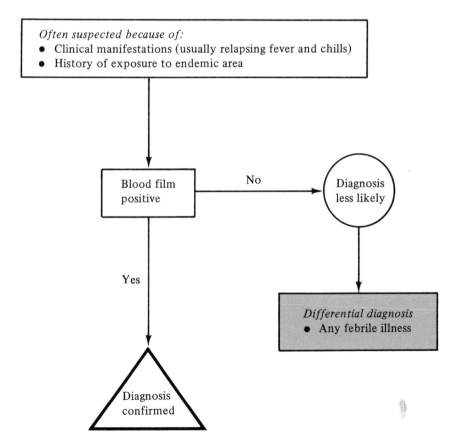

Often suspected because of:
- Clinical manifestations (usually relapsing fever and chills)
- History of exposure to endemic area

Blood film positive

No → Diagnosis less likely

Yes

Diagnosis confirmed

Differential diagnosis
- Any febrile illness

▶ **CLINICAL MANIFESTATIONS**

Primary—Prodrome of coryza, cough, followed by conjunctivitis, photophobia lymphadenopathy, and generalized maculopapular rash starting on the face and trunk and lasting approximately 4 days. Koplik spots may be seen on buccal mucosa.
Secondary—Pneumonia and postinfectious encephalitis.

▶ **EPIDEMIOLOGY**

Agent: Viral—rubeola virus.

Reservoir: Humans.

Transmission: Droplet spread, direct contact, or airborne spread of oropharyngeal secretions.

Incubation period: 7–14 days.

Period of communicability: 4 days prior to rash until 4 days after rash.

Duration of immunity: Lifelong.

▶ **DIAGNOSTIC PROCEDURES**

Cultures: Specimens—nasal and pharyngeal swabs.
  Media—tissue cultures.

Serology: Complement fixation.

Other: Multinucleated giant cells often seen in urine, sediment, and oropharyngeal scrapings early during illness.

▶ **MANAGEMENT**

Patient treatment: None.

Patient isolation: Keep home from school or work until 1 week after onset of rash. Respiratory isolation for hospitalized patients (see page 232).

Immunization: Live attenuated virus vaccine one dose for those age 15 months or older (see page 218).

Management of contacts: Susceptible close contacts should receive 0.25 ml/kg serum immune globulin, be isolated as above if they have upper respiratory symptoms, and be vaccinated 3 months later. *Note:* In epidemic situations, children 6–14 months old may be vaccinated but should be revaccinated after 15 months of age.

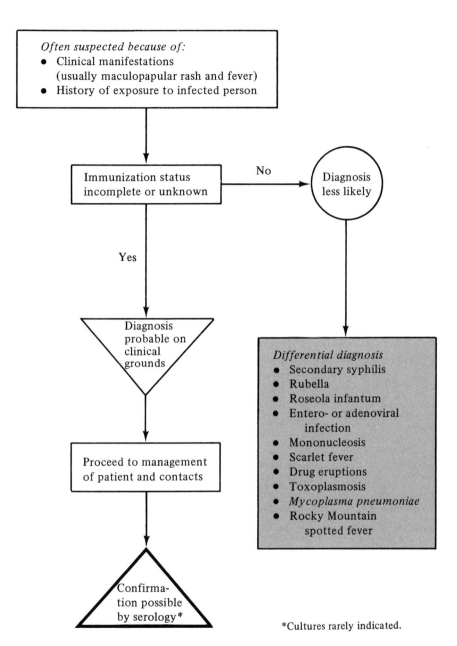

Often suspected because of:
- Clinical manifestations
  (usually maculopapular rash and fever)
- History of exposure to infected person

Immunization status
incomplete or unknown

No

Diagnosis
less likely

Yes

Diagnosis
probable on
clinical
grounds

Proceed to management
of patient and contacts

Differential diagnosis
- Secondary syphilis
- Rubella
- Roseola infantum
- Entero- or adenoviral
  infection
- Mononucleosis
- Scarlet fever
- Drug eruptions
- Toxoplasmosis
- *Mycoplasma pneumoniae*
- Rocky Mountain
  spotted fever

Confirma-
tion possible
by serology*

*Cultures rarely indicated.

▶ **CLINICAL MANIFESTATIONS**

1. Nasopharyngeal colonization usually asymptomatic.
2. Sepsis with sudden onset of fever, headache, nausea, vomiting, and a petechial rash. Occasionally septic arthritis and meningitis. Rarely pneumonia.

▶ **EPIDEMIOLOGY**

Agent: Bacterial—*Neisseria meningitidis;* serogroups A, B, C, most common.

Reservoir: Humans. Asymptomatic carriers are common (1–25% of civilian populations).

Transmission: Direct contact as well as contact with oral–nasal secretions of infected persons and asymptomatic carriers.

Incubation period: 2–10 days.

Period of communicability: While organisms present in nose and throat, and usually disappear within 24 hours after the onset of the appropriate antibiotic therapy.

Duration of immunity: Group-specific immunity of unknown duration.

▶ **DIAGNOSTIC PROCEDURES**

Cultures: Specimens—blood, spinal fluid, joint fluid, skin lesions. Nasopharyngeal cultures often misleading due to high carrier rate.
Media—modified Thayer-Martin agar.

Other: Gram-negative diplococci often seen on gram stain of specimens. Counter immunoelectrophoresis of CSF may help by demonstrating meningococcal polysaccharides.

▶ **MANAGEMENT**

Patient treatment: Crystalline sodium penicillin IV, 100,000 units/kg/day in 4 divided doses. Alternative drugs include chloramphenicol and sulfadiazine.

Patient isolation: Respiratory isolation (see page 232) until 24 hours after treatment is started.

Immunization: Vaccines against Group A and Group C exist, but should be reserved for use in *epidemic* situations.

Management of contacts: Check household contacts for symptoms of diseases within 48 hours after contact. Prophylactic antibiotics for intimate (household or mouth-to-mouth) contacts:

1. Rifampin x 2 days (if sensitivity of specific organism is not known): infants less than 1 year, 5 mg/kg every 12 hours. Children over 1 year, 10 mg/kg every 12 hours. Adults, 300 mg every 12 hours.

(Continued on next page)

MANAGEMENT (Cont.)

  2. Minocycline may be considered as alternative, but has more side effects, *or*
  3. Sulfadiazine x 2 days (*only* if specific organism known to be sensitive): children 0.5 gm PO q12h; adults, 1 gm PO q12h. *Note:* Penicillin and ampicillin are *not* effective for prophylaxis.

Other: Routine laundering of articles soiled with secretions may help limit spread.

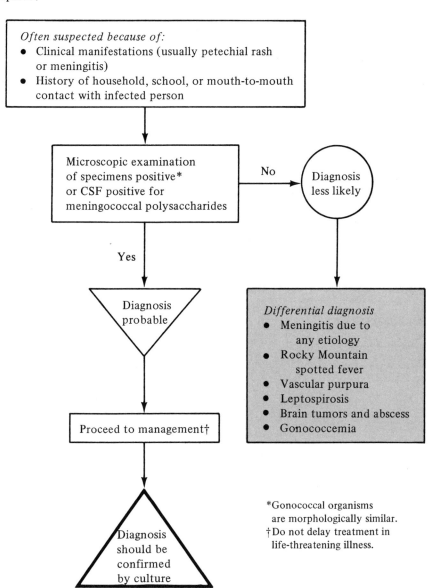

Often suspected because of:
  • Clinical manifestations (usually petechial rash or meningitis)
  • History of household, school, or mouth-to-mouth contact with infected person

Microscopic examination of specimens positive* or CSF positive for meningococcal polysaccharides

No → Diagnosis less likely

Yes

Diagnosis probable

Differential diagnosis
  • Meningitis due to any etiology
  • Rocky Mountain spotted fever
  • Vascular purpura
  • Leptospirosis
  • Brain tumors and abscess
  • Gonococcemia

Proceed to management†

Diagnosis should be confirmed by culture

*Gonococcal organisms are morphologically similar.
†Do not delay treatment in life-threatening illness.

▶ **CLINICAL MANIFESTATIONS**

Fever, lymphadenopathy, pharyngitis, and splenomegaly, with protracted malaise and fatigue. Jaundice and erythematous petechial rash of the hard palate may be observed. Course mild and difficult to diagnose or confirm in children under 5 years of age.

▶ **EPIDEMIOLOGY**

Agent: Viral—Epstein-Barr virus (herpes group virus).

Reservoir: Probably only humans.

Transmission: Usually by direct intimate contact or droplet spread.

Incubation period: 2–6 weeks.

Period of communicability: Unknown, but at least during acute illness.

Duration of immunity: Probably lifelong.

▶ **DIAGNOSTIC PROCEDURES**

Serology: Mono spot, a useful screening test.
    Heterophile antibody titers, positive within 2–4 weeks and decreases over several months. False positives seen in Hodgkins', sarcoidosis, SLE, hepatitis, lymphoma.
    EB virus antibody titers may be useful in heterophile-negative cases.

Other: Blood smear shows at least 10% abnormal lymphocytes (Dowdry cells) and a 20–40% lymphocytosis. Liver function tests (SGOT, SGPT, bilirubin, alkaline phosphotase) may be abnormal.

▶ **MANAGEMENT**

Patient treatment: None.

Patient isolation: Avoid sharing of saliva-contaminated articles (e.g., toothbrushes).

Other: Routine laundering of articles contaminated by nasal or pharyngeal secretions *may* be beneficial.

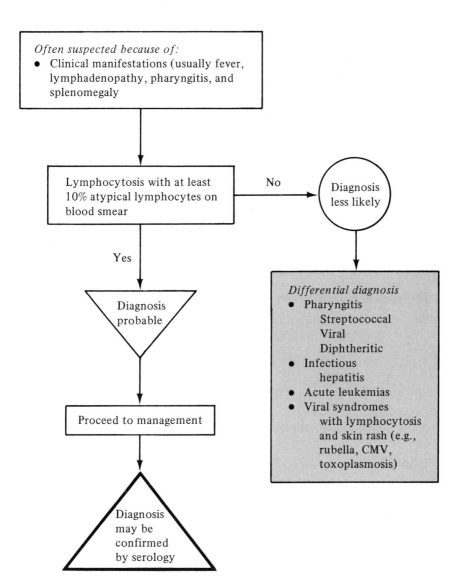

▶ CLINICAL MANIFESTATIONS

1. Malaise and low-grade fever followed in several days by painful, often bilateral salivary gland (usually parotid) swelling which lasts 6–10 days.
2. Mild viral meningoencephalitis common, pancreatitis, orchitis, oophoritis, and unilateral hearing loss not uncommon, and arthritis or myocarditis rare.

▶ EPIDEMIOLOGY

Agent: Viral—mumps virus.

Reservoir: Humans.

Transmission: Droplet spread and/or direct contact.

Incubation period: About 12–26 days, usually 18 days.

Period of communicability: From 1 week before swelling starts until it subsides.

Duration of immunity: Usually lifelong after infection or vaccination.

▶ DIAGNOSTIC PROCEDURES

Cultures: Specimens—saliva, blood, urine, or CSF.
       Media—tissue cultures (useful, but often not readily available).

Serology: A fourfold increase in C.F. titers indicates recent infection. A titer of less than 1 : 8 usually indicates susceptibility.

Skin tests: Available, but not reliable or diagnostic of acute disease.

Other: Clinical picture often adequate for diagnosis of acute infection, but elevated serum amylase may help.

▶ MANAGEMENT

Patient treatment: Symptomatic for pain and fever.

Patient isolation: Keep home from school or work until swelling subsides. If in hospital, respiratory isolation (see page 232).

Immunization: Live attenuated virus vaccine for children 15 months or older, and for nonimmune, nonpregnant young adults. Vaccine about 90% effective, and often available in combination with measles and rubella as MMR.

Management of contacts: Nonimmune household contacts might benefit from vaccine if given early. Consider mumps immune globulin or standard immune serum globulin for immunodeficient contacts.

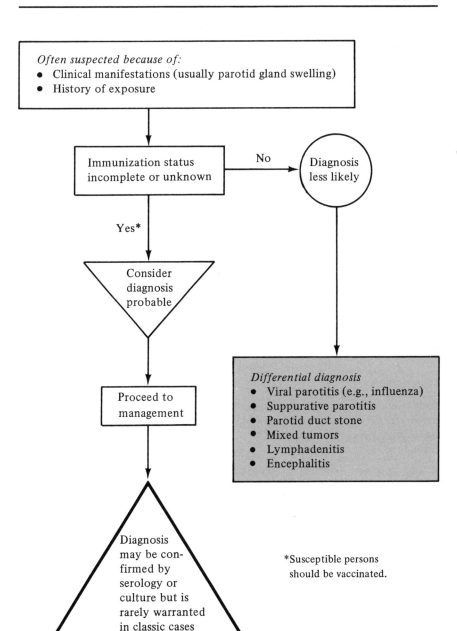

Often suspected because of:
- Clinical manifestations (usually parotid gland swelling)
- History of exposure

Immunization status incomplete or unknown

No → Diagnosis less likely

Yes*

Consider diagnosis probable

Proceed to management

Differential diagnosis
- Viral parotitis (e.g., influenza)
- Suppurative parotitis
- Parotid duct stone
- Mixed tumors
- Lymphadenitis
- Encephalitis

Diagnosis may be confirmed by serology or culture but is rarely warranted in classic cases

*Susceptible persons should be vaccinated.

▶ **CLINICAL MANIFESTATIONS**

1. Pruritic skin lesions, typically small, erythematous papules often found in hairy areas.
2. Body lice may rarely transmit rickettsial diseases. Excoriations and secondary infections.

▶ **EPIDEMIOLOGY**

Agent: Parasitic—three varieties of lice: *Pediculus humanis capitis* (head louse), *P. corporis* (body louse), *Phthirus pubis* (pubic or crab louse).

Reservoir: Humans.

Transmission: Direct contact with infected persons or contaminated articles like pillowcases, sheets, hats, and combs.

Incubation period: 1–4 weeks.

Period of communicability: Until lice and eggs are destroyed.

▶ **DIAGNOSTIC PROCEDURES**

Other: Search for lice (1–4 mm long depending on variety) and eggs ("nits" less than 1 mm, stuck to hair shafts).

▶ **MANAGEMENT**

Patient treatment: Gamma benzene hexachloride (Lindane, Kwell) topically. Treat again in 1 week. Alternatives include nonprescription insecticide preparations such as A-200 pyrinate. *Note:* Shaving of hair or combing out nits is unnecessary.

Patient isolation: Keep out of school until treatment applied.

Management of contacts: Examine for lice and eggs.

Other: Limit sharing of personal items such as hats, towels, and combs. Routine laundering of clothes and bedding at time of treatment.

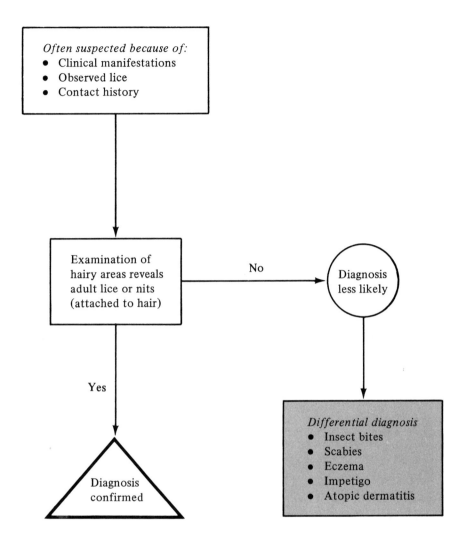

▶ **CLINICAL MANIFESTATIONS**

1. Catarrhal stage lasts 1–2 weeks, with nasal discharge, conjunctivitis, and mild cough without fever. Paroxysms of coughing ending in a loud crowing inspiration (whoop), production of thick sputum, occasional vomiting.
2. Bronchopneumonia, pulmonary atelectasis, eye or brain hemorrhage, rectal prolapse, and encephalopathy.

▶ **EPIDEMIOLOGY**

Agent: Bacterial—*Bordetella pertussis.*

Reservoir: Humans.

Transmission: By direct respiratory droplet spread, or by contact with articles contaminated by respiratory secretions.

Incubation period: 5–21 days, usually 1 week.

Period of communicability: As long as 4 weeks. Most infectious during catarrhal stage.

Duration of immunity: Possibly lifelong.

▶ **DIAGNOSTIC PROCEDURES**

Cultures: Specimens—throat or sputum.
　　　　　Media—Bordet-Gengou with penicillin.

Serology: Limited usefulness. Agglutination titers of value only late in the disease. Fluorescent antibody techniques experimentally available, and may help make rapid diagnosis.

Other: Lymphocytoses common.

▶ **MANAGEMENT**

Patient treatment: Erythromycin 30–50 mg/kg/day in 4 doses PO, IM, or IV x 10 days. Alternate drug ampicillin. Mild sedation with barbiturates may relieve paroxysms.

Patient isolation: Keep away from young children for 4 weeks. If in hospital, respiratory isolation (see page 232).

Immunization: DTP (diphtheria and tetanus toxoids plus pertussis vaccine) recommended at 2, 4, 6, and 18 months and again at 5 years.

Management of contacts: Give DTP boosters x 1 and erythromycin (or ampicillin) for 10 days to contacts under 4 years of age, regardless of immune status.

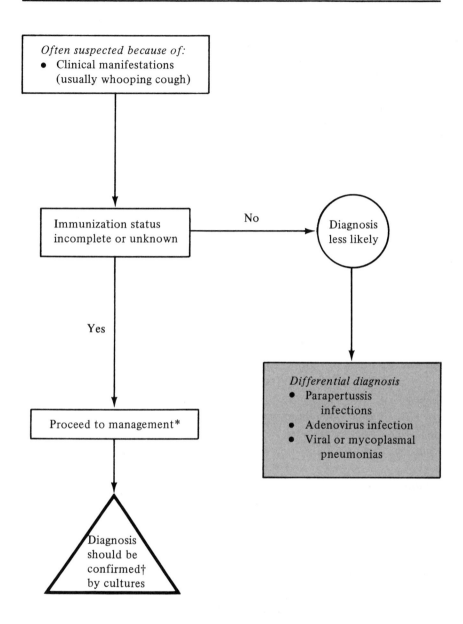

*Obtain cultures before starting antibiotic.
†Culturing of contacts may increase chances of isolating organisms.

▶ **CLINICAL MANIFESTATIONS**

1. The original site of infection (bubo) becomes inflamed. Painful lymphadenitis and fever follow.
2. Septicemia, petechial hemorrhages, shock, coma, meningitis, and pneumonia are common.

▶ **EPIDEMIOLOGY**

Agent: Bacterial—*Yersinia pestis.*

Reservoir: Rodents.

Transmission: By infected rodent fleas or by direct contact with the tissues of an infected animal. Patients with plague pneumonia may transmit infection by droplet spread.

Incubation period: Usually 2–6 days in bubonic plague, and 1–4 days in pneumonia plague.

Period of communicability: Only during active pneumonia, if present.

Duration of immunity: Limited and variable.

▶ **DIAGNOSTIC PROCEDURES**

Cultures: Specimens—pus, sputum, and blood.
        Media—blood agar plates for pus and sputum, nutrient broth for blood.

Serology: Passive hemagglutination, complement fixation, or immunoelectrophoretic agar-gel precipitation techniques are useful.

Other: Microscopic examination of specimen stained with fluorescent antiserum allows rapid identification.

▶ **MANAGEMENT**

Patient treatment: Hospitalize all patients. Streptomycin, tetracycline, or chloramphenicol are the most effective drugs. Sulfonamides may be used if other drugs are unavailable. Penicillin is *not* effective.

Patient isolation: Strict isolation (see page 232) only if pneumonia is present. Assure that fleas in clothing are destroyed.

Immunization: Consider only for those working with infected animals, or traveling to rural Vietnam, Cambodia, or Laos.

Management of contacts: Disinfect with insecticide powders and observe 10 days for symptoms. Contacts of plague pneumonia should also have daily temperature readings and chemoprophylaxis (streptomycin, tetracycline, chloramphenicol, or a sulfa).

Other: Control of rats and other wild rodents. Flea dusting of wild animals.

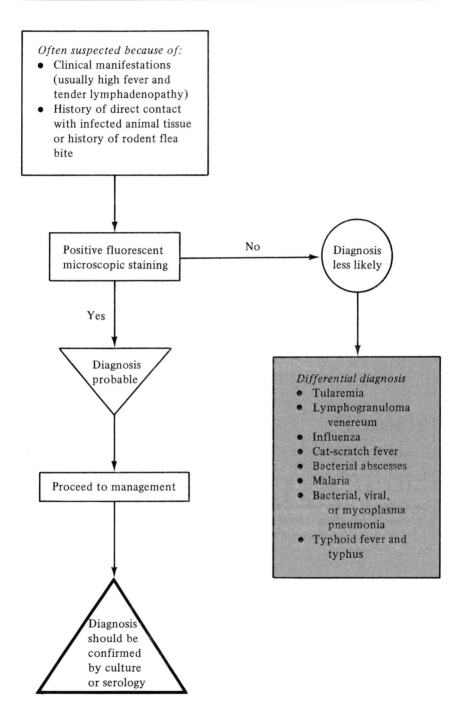

Often suspected because of:
- Clinical manifestations (usually high fever and tender lymphadenopathy)
- History of direct contact with infected animal tissue or history of rodent flea bite

Positive fluorescent microscopic staining

No → Diagnosis less likely

Yes

Diagnosis probable

Proceed to management

Diagnosis should be confirmed by culture or serology

Differential diagnosis
- Tularemia
- Lymphogranuloma venereum
- Influenza
- Cat-scratch fever
- Bacterial abscesses
- Malaria
- Bacterial, viral, or mycoplasma pneumonia
- Typhoid fever and typhus

▶ **CLINICAL MANIFESTATIONS**

Commonly pneumonia, meningitis, otitis, or peritonitis.

▶ **EPIDEMIOLOGY**

Agent: Bacterial—*Streptococcus pneumoniae,* numerous serotypes.

Reservoir: Humans.

Transmission: By direct contact, droplet spread, or indirectly by contaminated articles.

Incubation period: Not well determined, probably several days.

Period of communicability: Duration of presence of organism.

Duration of immunity: Serotype specific. About 80% of disease is caused by 12 serotypes.

▶ **DIAGNOSTIC PROCEDURES**

Cultures: Specimen—depends on site.
        Media—blood agar.

Serology: Not clinically useful.

Other: Gram staining useful (gram-positive lancet-shaped diplococci). Neufeld guellung or capsular precipitation reaction techniques may help identify serotypes. CIE of CSF may help in diagnosis of meningitis.

▶ **MANAGEMENT**

Patient treatment: Penicillin, erythromycin, or cephalosporin. *Note:* Some strains are penicillin-resistant.

Patient isolation: Unnecessary.

Immunization: Vaccine only recommended for high-risk patients over 2 years of age (asplenia, chronic metabolic, pulmonary or cardiac disease). See page 221.

Other measures: Avoid overcrowding in living quarters whenever practical.

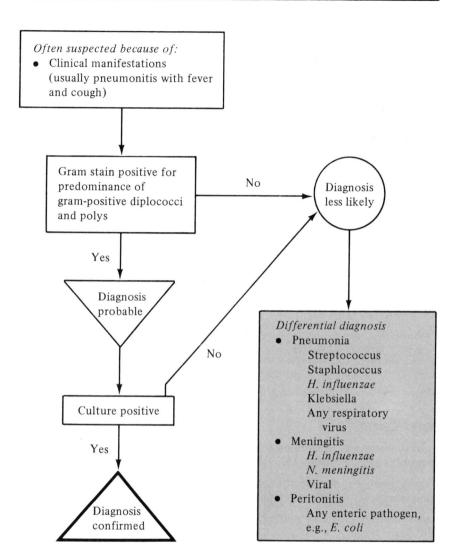

Often suspected because of:
- Clinical manifestations (usually pneumonitis with fever and cough)

Gram stain positive for predominance of gram-positive diplococci and polys

No → Diagnosis less likely

Yes

Diagnosis probable

No

Culture positive

Yes

Diagnosis confirmed

Differential diagnosis
- Pneumonia
    Streptococcus
    Staphlococcus
    H. influenzae
    Klebsiella
    Any respiratory
    virus
- Meningitis
    H. influenzae
    N. meningitis
    Viral
- Peritonitis
    Any enteric pathogen,
    e.g., *E. coli*

▶ CLINICAL MANIFESTATIONS

1. Usually asymptomatic or mild infection with flu-like symptoms of nausea, vomiting, diarrhea, meningeal irritation, and myalgias.
2. Muscular weakness may progress to paralysis (usually asymmetrical and flaccid).

▶ EPIDEMIOLOGY

Agent: Viral—polio virus, serotypes 1, 2, and 3.

Reservoir: Humans.

Transmission: Direct person-to-person contact by fecal-oral and pharyngeal-oropharyngeal routes.

Incubation period: 3–35 days.

Period of communicability: Up to 6 weeks or longer.

Duration of immunity: Lifelong serotype immunity.

▶ DIAGNOSTIC PROCEDURES

Cultures: Specimen—pharyngeal and stool.
　　　　　　Media—tissue culture.

Serology: Neutralizing or complement fixing antibody titer elevation.

Other: Abnormal CSF including leukocytosis and elevated protein.

▶ MANAGEMENT

Patient treatment: Symptomatic treatment of noncomplicated cases, supportive treatment of paralytic disease.

Patient isolation: Not practical due to prevalence of asymptomatic infection in community. If in hospital, enteric precautions (see page 233).

Immunization: Trivalent oral polio vaccine at 2, 4, 6 months, 1-1/2 years, and 4-6 years.

Management of contacts: Isolation and vaccination of nonimmunized contacts.

Other: If two or more cases with identical serotypes are reported from a community within a 4-week period, immunize the community.

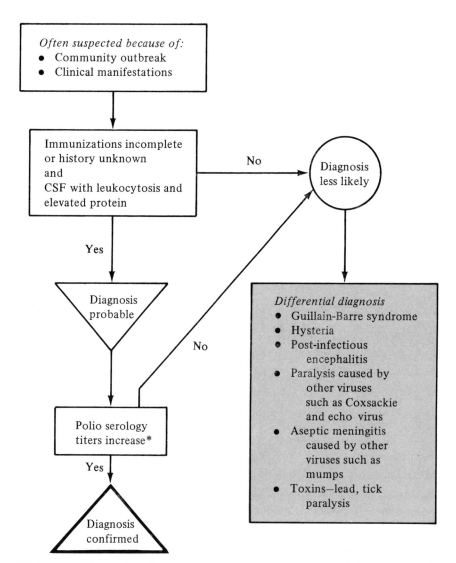

*Cultures may also confirm diagnosis and are critical for differentiating "wild" from vaccine-associated disease.

▶ **CLINICAL MANIFESTATIONS**

1. Sensory changes around the wound, headache, fever, photophobia, paralysis, and muscle spasms causing inability to swallow.
2. Almost always fatal with laryngospasm and respiratory paralysis within 1 week.

▶ **EPIDEMIOLOGY**

Agent: Viral—rabies virus.

Reservoir: Wild or domestic animals including bats, skunks, foxes, mongooses, dogs, cats, and raccoons.

Transmission: By saliva of rabid animal entering the skin (via bite or scratch).

Incubation period: Depends on site and size of inoculum. Usually 2–8 weeks, occasionally as long as 1 year.

Period of communicability: Variable. Depends on species.

Duration of immunity: Variable. For pre-exposure protection, give boosters at least every 3 years.

▶ **DIAGNOSTIC PROCEDURES**

Cultures: Specimens—saliva, urine, CSF, salivary glands, brain.
          Media—tissue cultures and/or mouse inoculation.

Serology: Complement fixation titers are useful.

Other: For rapid identification (in all animal species) use fluorescent antibody staining of corneal impressions, mucosal scrapings, or *brain tissue*. Negri bodies are often found in brain tissue.

▶ **MANAGEMENT**

Patient treatment: Intensive, supportive medical care with special attention to major neurologic, pituitary, pulmonary, and cardiovascular complications.

Patient isolation: Strict isolation (see page 232) for patients. Suspected rabid animals should be handled only by trained, immunized people.

Immunization: Pre-exposure—two 1-ml doses of DEV (duck embryo vaccine) subcutaneously given 1 month apart. Give booster 6 months later and then every 2–3 years. Test serology 1 month after each booster. For veterinarians and repeatedly exposed sanitarians and laboratory personnel only.
Post-exposure—follow indications on page 81. Antiserum (see page 221) *plus* 21 daily doses of DEV. Two boosters 10 and 20 days after initial series. Repeat boosters monthly till serology is positive.

Management of contacts: Follow guide on page 80.

(Continued on next page)

► **MANAGEMENT (Cont.)**

Other measures

1. Animal rabies is best controlled by vaccination of dogs and cats, elimination of stray animals or "exotic" pets (e.g., raccoons) and reduction of reservoir pests (e.g., mongoose in Puerto Rico).
2. Immediate washing of bite wounds with soap and water is very effective in preventing rabies.

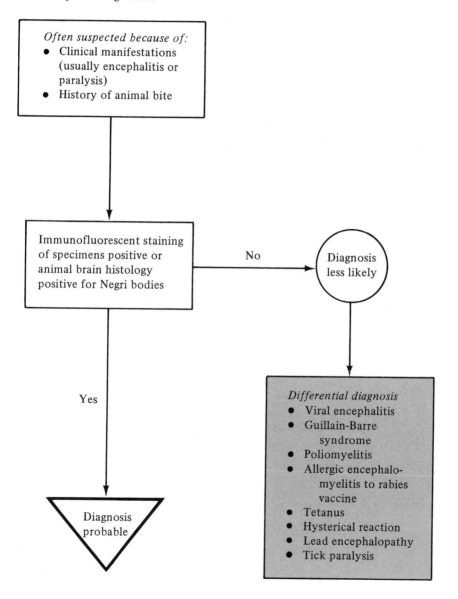

Often suspected because of:
- Clinical manifestations (usually encephalitis or paralysis)
- History of animal bite

Immunofluorescent staining of specimens positive or animal brain histology positive for Negri bodies

No → Diagnosis less likely

Yes

Diagnosis probable

Differential diagnosis
- Viral encephalitis
- Guillain-Barre syndrome
- Poliomyelitis
- Allergic encephalomyelitis to rabies vaccine
- Tetanus
- Hysterical reaction
- Lead encephalopathy
- Tick paralysis

▶ **QUESTIONS TO ASK IN DECIDING
WHETHER OR NOT TO ADMINISTER
POST-EXPOSURE RABIES PROPHYLAXIS**

(Use as rough guide only. Consult your health department.)

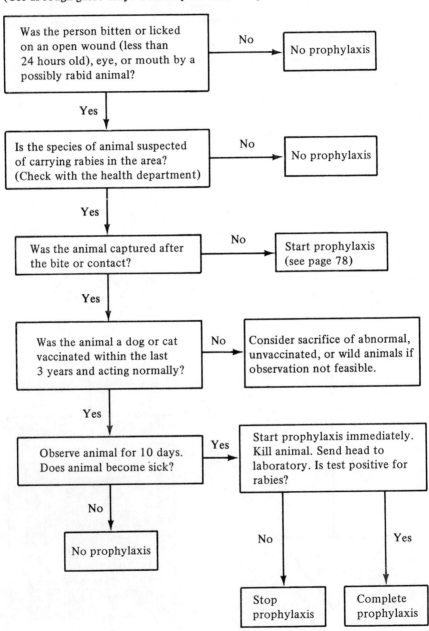

POST-EXPOSURE ANTIRABIES GUIDE

The following recommendations are only a guide. They should be used in conjunction with knowledge of the animal species involved, circumstances of the bite or other exposure, vaccination status of the animal, and presence of rabies in the region.

Animal and Its Condition		*Treatment*	
		Kind of exposure	
Species	*Condition at time of attack*	*Bite*	*Nonbite* *
WILD			
Skunk			
Fox			
Raccoon	Regard as rabid	$S + V^a$	$S + V^a$
Bat			
Mongoose			
DOMESTIC			
Dog	Healthy	None [b]	None [b]
	Escaped (unknown)	$S + V$	V^c
Cat	Rabid	$S + V^a$	$S + V^a$
OTHER	Consider individually		

* Scratches, abrasions, or open wounds.
V   Rabies Vaccine (duck embryo vaccine, DEV).
S   Antirabies serum (rabies immune globulin, RIG). Give 20 IU human RIG or 40 IU equine RIG. (½ in wound and ½ IM).
[a] Discontinue vaccine if fluorescent antibody (FA) tests of animal killed at time of attack are negative.
[b] Begin S + V at first sign of rabies in biting dog or cat during holding period (10 days).
[c] 14 doses of DEV.

▶ **CLINICAL MANIFESTATIONS**

1. Almost 30% of infections asymptomatic. Occasional headaches and conjunctivitis, then fever, postauricular lymphadenopathy, arthralgias, and a diffuse, macular rash usually lasting 3 days.
2. Infants with congenital rubella syndrome may have jaundice, hepatosplenomegaly, thrombocytopenia, cataracts, retinopathy, congenital heart disease, microcephaly and deafness. (TORCHES' syndrome seen in infants with toxoplasmosis, rubella, CMV, herpes, and syphilis.)

▶ **EPIDEMIOLOGY**

Agent: Viral—rubella.

Reservoir: Humans.

Transmission: By direct or indirect contact with droplets, secretions, blood, urine, or feces of patients. Transplacentally in congenital rubella.

Incubation period: 2–3 weeks.

Period of communicability: From 1 week before to 1 week after skin rash has appeared. Infants born with congenital rubella syndrome may shed virus for several years.

Duration of immunity: Usually lifelong after infection or vaccination.

▶ **DIAGNOSTIC PROCEDURES**

Cultures: Specimens—throat, blood, and urine. (Also CSF and other tissues in congenital infection.)
Media—tissue culture. Not as useful as serology.

Serology: Hemagglutination inhibition (HI) titers. Increasing titers indicate recent infection. Persistent titers of 1 : 4 or more indicate immunity (see page 000). Congenital infections can be confirmed by specific IgM rubella antibodies, or IgG antibodies persisting past 6 months.

▶ **MANAGEMENT**

Patient treatment: Symptomatic.

Patient isolation: Only to protect susceptible pregnant women. If in hospital, strict isolation (see page 232).

Immunization: Live, attenuated virus vaccine, one dose for those age 15 months or older (see page 218).

Management of contacts: Any pregnant female exposed to rubella should have serological evaluation for the presence of immunity. If she is not immune, repeated titers and close observation for the disease should be carried out. Immune serum globulin is of no proven value and interferes with serological monitoring. Pregnant women acquiring disease during the first trimester should consider abortion.

(Continued on next page)

▶ MANAGEMENT (Cont.)

Other: For postpubertal or "impregnable" females and personnel working with pregnant women, check immunological status if unknown and if serology negative, vaccinate if contraception can be assured for 3 months after vaccination. (Immediately postpartum for pregnant females.)

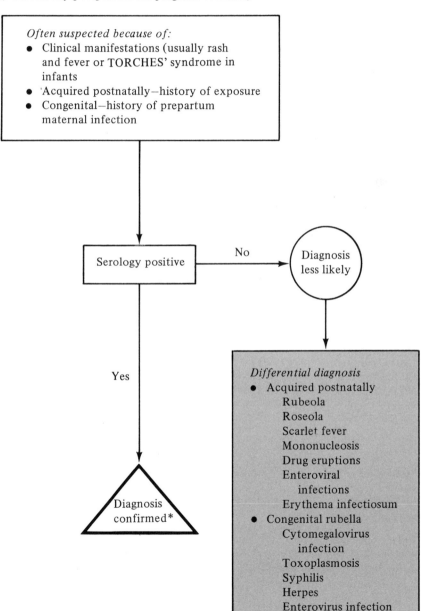

Often suspected because of:
- Clinical manifestations (usually rash and fever or TORCHES' syndrome in infants
- Acquired postnatally—history of exposure
- Congenital—history of prepartum maternal infection

Serology positive

No → Diagnosis less likely

Yes

Diagnosis confirmed*

Differential diagnosis
- Acquired postnatally
  Rubeola
  Roseola
  Scarlet fever
  Mononucleosis
  Drug eruptions
  Enteroviral infections
  Erythema infectiosum
- Congenital rubella
  Cytomegalovirus infection
  Toxoplasmosis
  Syphilis
  Herpes
  Enterovirus infection

*Culture confirmation is rarely needed.

▶ **CLINICAL MANIFESTATIONS**

1. Gastroenteritis with sudden onset of diarrhea, often with abdominal pain, nausea, vomiting, and fever.
2. Bacteremia rarely leading to abscess formation or subsequent osteomyelitis, arthritis, cholecystitis, endocarditis, or meningitis. (For typhoid fever, see page 110.)

▶ **EPIDEMIOLOGY**

Agent: Bacterial—numerous salmonella serogroups.

Reservoir: Domestic animals, particularly cattle, poultry and their eggs, turtles, and humans. Long-term carriers are rare.

Transmission: Fecal-oral route by direct person-to-person or animal-to-person transmission, or by consumption of contaminated food or drink.

Incubation period: 6–72 hours.

Period of communicability: Days to several weeks.

▶ **DIAGNOSTIC PROCEDURES**

Cultures: Specimens—stool and blood (if bacteremia suspected).
　　　　　Note: Serotyping of the organism is important for tracing the source of infection.
　　　　　Media—tetrathionate enrichment broth or SS agar.

Serology: Not helpful (see typhoid fever, page 110).

Other: Stool smear usually shows numerous polys.

▶ **MANAGEMENT**

Patient treatment: Antibiotic treatment of gastroenteritis is unnecessary and may prolong the carrier state. Prevention of dehydration is important. Severe, chronic, or systemic infections should be treated with ampicillin or chloramphenicol.

Patient isolation: Enteric precautions (see page 233) and restrictions as for contacts.

Management of contacts: Household contacts and patients should be restricted from commercial food handling and care of children or debilitated persons until three daily stool cultures are negative (start after antibiotics have been completed).

Other: Encourage prompt refrigeration of foods in small quantities. Discourage consumption of raw eggs and long-standing, nonrefrigerated foods. Commercially used refrigerators should be routinely checked for adequate functioning.

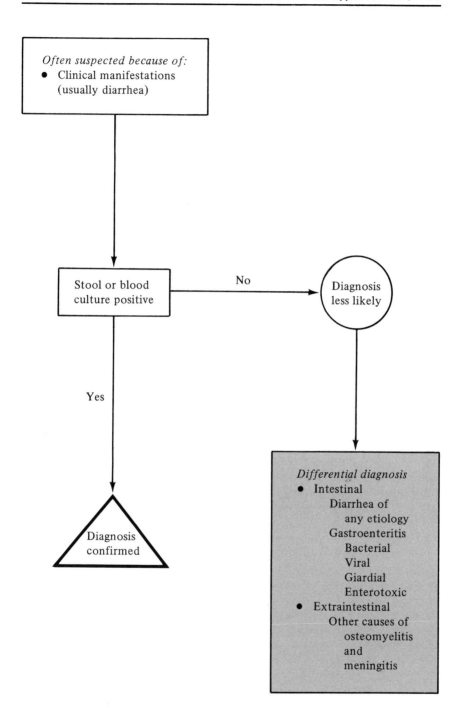

Often suspected because of:
- Clinical manifestations
  (usually diarrhea)

Stool or blood culture positive

No

Diagnosis less likely

Yes

Diagnosis confirmed

Differential diagnosis
- Intestinal
    Diarrhea of
      any etiology
    Gastroenteritis
      Bacterial
      Viral
      Giardial
      Enterotoxic
- Extraintestinal
    Other causes of
      osteomyelitis
      and
      meningitis

▶ CLINICAL MANIFESTATIONS

1. Vesicles, papules, and linear "burrows" associated with intense itching. Common sites of infestations are intradigital, periumbilical, the "belt line," and the genital area.
2. Excoriations and bacterial superinfection.

Note: Scabies often imitates other lesions.

▶ EPIDEMIOLOGY

Agent: Arthropodic—a mite, *Sarcoptes scabiei.*

Reservoir: Humans. Animal mites can cause brief infestations in humans.

Transmission: Usually by direct contact from person to person, but may occur by contact with contaminated clothing or bedding.

Incubation period: Several days to weeks.

Period of communicability: As long as the ova and mites are present in skin.

▶ DIAGNOSTIC PROCEDURES

Other: The mite may be teased out of the burrow and identified microscopically.

▶ MANAGEMENT

Patient treatment: Gamma benzene hexachloride (e.g., Lindane, Kwell), or 10% crotamiton; applied topically. Reapplication in 7 days may be necessary. *Note:* Itching may persist several days after adequate treatment.

Patient isolation: None.

Management of contacts: None, but other household members are often infested. Casual contacts should be treated only if lesions are demonstrated.

Other: Routine laundering of clothing and bedding is recommended at time of treatment.

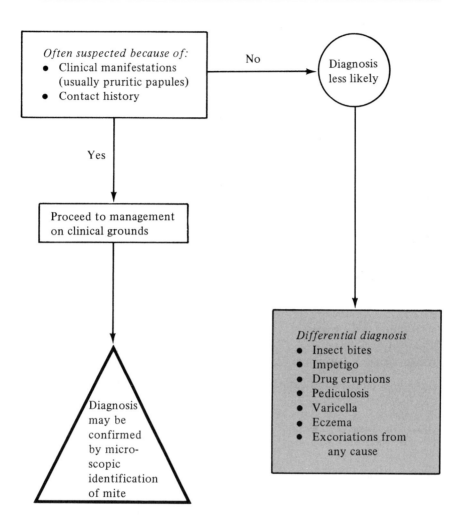

Often suspected because of:
- Clinical manifestations (usually pruritic papules)
- Contact history

No

Diagnosis less likely

Yes

Proceed to management on clinical grounds

Diagnosis may be confirmed by microscopic identification of mite

Differential diagnosis
- Insect bites
- Impetigo
- Drug eruptions
- Pediculosis
- Varicella
- Eczema
- Excoriations from any cause

▶ **CLINICAL MANIFESTATIONS**

1. Often asymptomatic.
2. Skin penetration by larvae results in dermatitis with pruritus and maculo-papular lesions.
3. Increasing parasite load may cause high spiking fevers, cough, abdominal pain, bloody diarrhea, urticaria, lymphadenopathy, and hepatomegaly.

▶ **EPIDEMIOLOGY**

Agent: Parasitic—the blood fluke (trematode) *Schistosoma mansoni* (South America, Caribbean, Africa). *S. hematobium* (Middle East) and *S. japonicum* (Asia) will not be covered here. Bird and rodent schistosome cercariae in bathing waters cause "swimmer's itch," a transient dermatitis.

Reservoir: Humans (for *S. mansoni*).

Transmission: By skin penetration of parasite larvae in stool-contaminated waters, where snails are an intermediate host.

Incubation period: 4–6 weeks after skin penetration.

Period of communicability: Not transmitted person to person. Ova may be present in stools for years.

▶ **DIAGNOSTIC PROCEDURES**

Serology: Complement fixation titers rarely useful, not confirmatory.

Skin test: Intradermal tests are not useful clinically.

Other: Examine stool specimens for ova. Rectal biopsies useful. Abnormal liver-function tests and eosinophilia (early in disease) often present.

▶ **MANAGEMENT**

Patient treatment: Asymptomatic or mild disease need not be treated since most effective drugs are toxic. First choice is sodium antimony dimercaptosuccinate (Astiban) 8 mg/kg/day IM x 5 days, or niridazole.

Patient isolation: None.

Management of contacts: None, but household members are often infected.

Other: Proper disposal of human excrement, purification of water supplies, education of public to avoid drinking or bathing in contaminated waters, eradication of snails in endemic areas, and concrete lining of irrigation ditches.

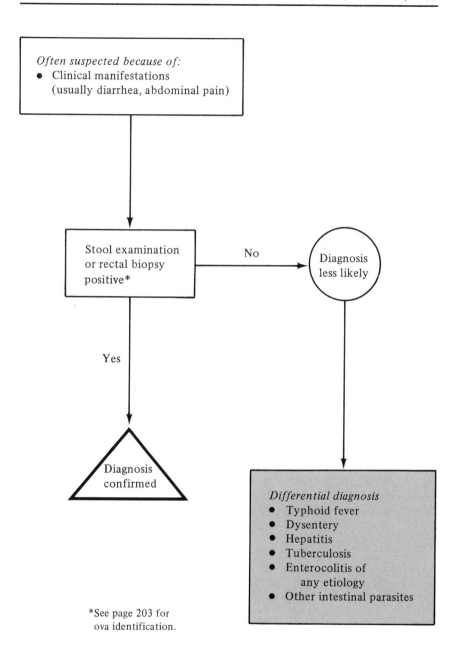

Often suspected because of:
- Clinical manifestations
  (usually diarrhea, abdominal pain)

Stool examination or rectal biopsy positive*

No → Diagnosis less likely

Yes

Diagnosis confirmed

Differential diagnosis
- Typhoid fever
- Dysentery
- Hepatitis
- Tuberculosis
- Enterocolitis of
  any etiology
- Other intestinal parasites

*See page 203 for
ova identification.

▶ **CLINICAL MANIFESTATIONS**

1. Acute onset of diarrhea, fever, abdominal pain, and cramps, often with nausea, vomiting, and headaches. Stools may contain pus, increased mucus, and blood.
2. Dehydration and circulatory collapse may occur.

▶ **EPIDEMIOLOGY**

Agent: Bacterial–Shigella spp. (*S. dysenteriae, S. flexneri, S. boydii,* and *S. sonnei* most common).

Reservoir: Humans.

Transmission: By direct or indirect fecal-oral transmission from patient or carrier, and by consumption of contaminated water, milk, and food.

Incubation period: 7 hours to 7 days, usually 3–4 days.

Period of communicability: As long as the person excretes bacteria, usually 1–4 weeks, but may be more than 1 year.

Duration of immunity: Some serotype specific immunity may develop.

▶ **DIAGNOSTIC PROCEDURES**

Cultures: Specimens–stool or rectal swab. Blood cultures are of little value.
        Media–TCBS or SS agar.

Serology: Not useful.

Other: White and red blood cells in the stool are suggestive of Shigella.

▶ **MANAGEMENT**

Patient treatment: Antibiotic therapy is usually not required. Ampicillin is recommended for severe adult cases and all sick infants. Alternatives include: trimethoprim-sulfa and tetracycline. Fluid and electrolyte therapy important.

Patient isolation: Enteric precautions (see page 233), and same restrictions as for management of contacts.

Management of contacts: Household contacts and patients should be excluded from food handling and the care of young children during the period of contact or illness and until three daily consecutive stool cultures are negative.

Other: Handwashing after defecation and sanitary disposal of human excrement. Protection of water supplies.

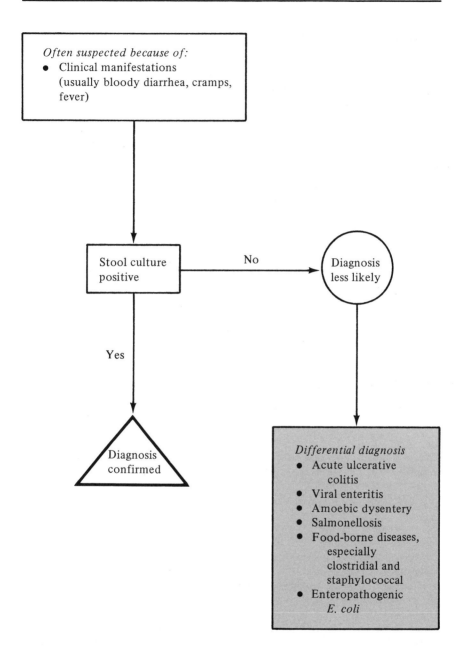

Often suspected because of:
- Clinical manifestations
  (usually bloody diarrhea, cramps,
  fever)

Stool culture positive

No → Diagnosis less likely

Yes

Diagnosis confirmed

Differential diagnosis
- Acute ulcerative colitis
- Viral enteritis
- Amoebic dysentery
- Salmonellosis
- Food-borne diseases, especially clostridial and staphylococcal
- Enteropathogenic E. coli

▶ CLINICAL MANIFESTATIONS

1. Boils, abscesses, surgical wound infections.
2. Impetigo (classically bullous) often in combination with group A strepto-cocci as the primary pathogen.
3. Osteomyelitis, meningitis, pneumonia, endocarditis, sepsis.
4. Mastitis in nursing mothers.
5. Scalded skin syndrome in infants.

▶ EPIDEMIOLOGY

Agent: Bacterial—various strains (phage types) of coagulase positive *Staphylo-coccus aureus.* Coagulase negative *S. epidermidis* may cause disease in compromised host.

Reservoir: Humans (partcularly skin and anterior nares).

Transmission: By contact with lesions of patients, or nasal discharge of carriers. One third of people are nasal carriers, and may contaminate food or other objects as well as infect themselves.

Incubation period: Variable, but usually about 1 week.

Period of communicability: As long as organisms are present in lesion or discharge.

Duration of immunity: None, but increasing age offers some resistance.

▶ DIAGNOSTIC PROCEDURES

Cultures: Specimens—swabs of skin lesions, anterior nares, blood, or other sites.
Media—blood agar.

Other: Phage-typing and antibiotic-resistance patterns often help in outbreak investigations. Gram-stains of specimens may be very useful.

▶ MANAGEMENT

Patient treatment: Impetigo can often be treated with local washing and peni-cillin (best is 600,000–1.2 million units benzathine IM). Erythromycin is good for penicillin-allergic patients and is effective against many community-acquired strains of staphylococci.
Previously treated or hospital acquired staphylococci are usually penicillin re-sistant: Use cloxacillin PO, dicloxacillin PO or methicillin IV or IM (severe infections).
Nasal carriers are difficult to treat. Treat only if their strain of organism is responsible for outbreaks. Treat with bacitracin, gentamicin, or neomycin oint-ment applied qid to the anterior nares for 2 weeks.

Patient isolation: If in hospital with pneumonia or enterocolitis, strict isola-tion (page 232); or with draining lesions, wound and skin precautions (page 233). For all infected infants in nursery, use strict isolation (page 232).

(Continued on next page)

▶ MANAGEMENT (Cont.)

Management of contacts: In nursery outbreaks, infant contacts should be cohort-isolated until discharge, with surveillance after discharge. Culture personnel.

Other: Investigate clusters of cases for common source (case, carrier, food, etc.). Exclude from work until treated persons with open lesions who are employed in nurseries, hospitals, or commercial food handling (see food poisoning, page 120). Careful aseptic techniques for surgery, IM injections, and IV therapy, and the limited use of antibiotics can help prevent infections.

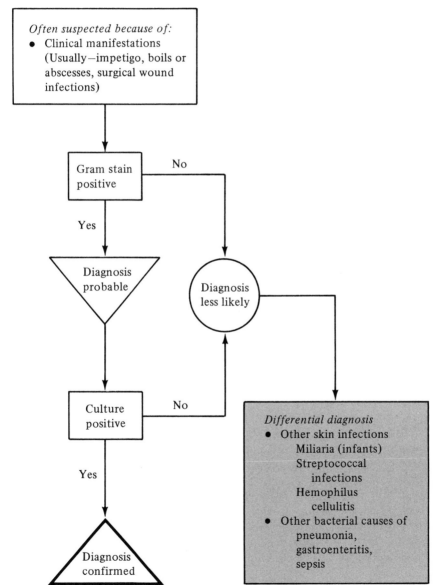

▶ **CLINICAL MANIFESTATIONS**

1. Pharyngitis—fever, sore throat, exudative tonsillitis, and tender cervical adenopathy. Asymptomatic carriers are prevalent.
2. Scarlet fever—same as above and including erythematous macular rash.
3. Impetigo or pyoderma—a usually superficial infection proceeding through vesicular, pustular, and encrusted stages.
4. Erysipelas—an acute cellulitis associated with tenderness and fever.
5. Puerperal fever—endometritis, sometimes associated with bacteremia, in postpartum or postabortion patients.
6. Neonatal meningitis and sepsis, endocarditis, urinary tract infections, and surgical wound infections.
7. Nonsuppurative complications of rheumatic fever or glomerulonephritis.

▶ **EPIDEMIOLOGY**

Agent: Bacterial—any one of various groups of beta hemolytic streptococci, usually group A (*S. pyogenes*).

Reservoir: Humans.

Transmission: Usually by direct droplet spread from a patient or carrier. Occasionally by ingesting contaminated foods.

Incubation period: 1–5 days.

Period of communicability: Untreated cases 10–20 days; treated cases 24 hours.

Duration of immunity: Of little significance, since immunity is only type-specific.

▶ **DIAGNOSTIC PROCEDURES**

Cultures: Specimen—sites as indicated (culture swabs can be sent dry, without transport media).
  Media—blood agar (rabbit or sheep).

Serology: A fourfold rise in streptozyme titers, or a single titer of at least 1 : 400, confirms recent infection.

Other: Immunofluorescent techniques are available for rapid identification of bacteria in culture material.

▶ **MANAGEMENT**

Patient treatment: A single IM dose of benzathine penicillin G is the best treatment for pharyngitis, scarlet fever, impetigo, and erysipelas (600,000 units for children weighing less than 30 kg, 1.2 million units for those over 30 kg. For neonatal dosage see page 152). Alternative treatments include 10 days of oral penicillin or erythromycin, (IV antibiotics for more severe infections). Rheumatic heart disease prophylaxis, see page 175.

Patient isolation: Keep home from school/work for 24 hours after onset of treatment.

(Continued on next page)

▶ MANAGEMENT (Cont.)

Management of contacts: If in hospital, isolation depends on site of infection (see page 232). Culture household contacts and treat if symptomatic.

Other: Infected commercial food handlers should not work while infectious. Discourage consumption of nonboiled, nonpasteurized milk. Encourage prompt refrigeration of prepared foods in small quantities. Assure use of sterile technique during surgical and obstetrical procedures.

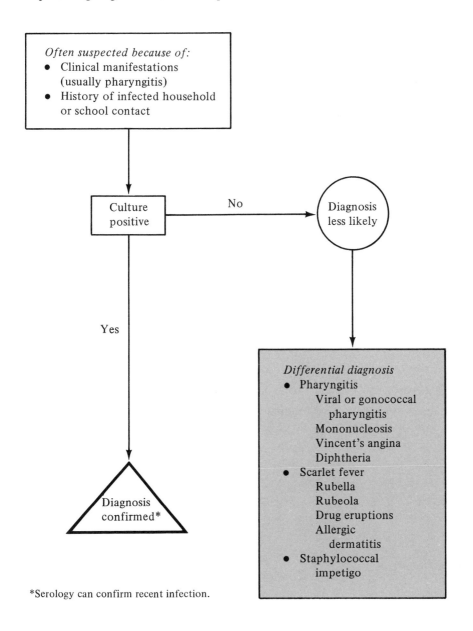

Often suspected because of:
- Clinical manifestations (usually pharyngitis)
- History of infected household or school contact

Culture positive

No → Diagnosis less likely

Yes

Diagnosis confirmed*

Differential diagnosis
- Pharyngitis
  Viral or gonococcal pharyngitis
  Mononucleosis
  Vincent's angina
  Diphtheria
- Scarlet fever
  Rubella
  Rubeola
  Drug eruptions
  Allergic dermatitis
- Staphylococcal impetigo

*Serology can confirm recent infection.

▶ **CLINICAL MANIFESTATIONS**

1. Often asymptomatic.
2. Abdominal pain, nausea, vomiting, diarrhea, weight loss, and weakness. Severity dependent on parasite load in the small instestine. Immunosuppressed patients may develop "hyperinfection."
3. Dermatitis and cough may develop while the larvae first penetrate the skin or pass through the lungs in their migration to the GI tract.

▶ **EPIDEMIOLOGY**

Agent: A parasite, the nematode *Strongyloides stercoralis.*

Reservoir: Humans.

Transmission: By skin contact, usually bare feet, with soil contaminated with human feces. Possibly by consumption of contaminated food.

Incubation period: About 2 weeks from time of larvae penetration of skin until new larvae appear in stools.

Period of communicability: Indefinite, as long as larvae present in stools. Not transmitted directly person to person.

▶ **DIAGNOSTIC PROCEDURES**

Serology: Filarial CF titers usually positive, but not clinically useful.

Other: Microscopic examination of fresh stool or duodenal aspirate for larvae. Eosinophilia commonly present.

▶ **MANAGEMENT**

Patient treatment: Thiabendazole (Mintezol) 25 mg/kg PO bid x 2 days is recommended for all those infested, because of danger of "hyperinfection." Repeated treatment in 1 week. Pyrvinium pamoate (Povan) is alternate.

Patient isolation: None.

Management of contacts: None. Check stools of household members for larvae.

Other: Sanitary disposal of human feces and wearing shoes are the best control methods.

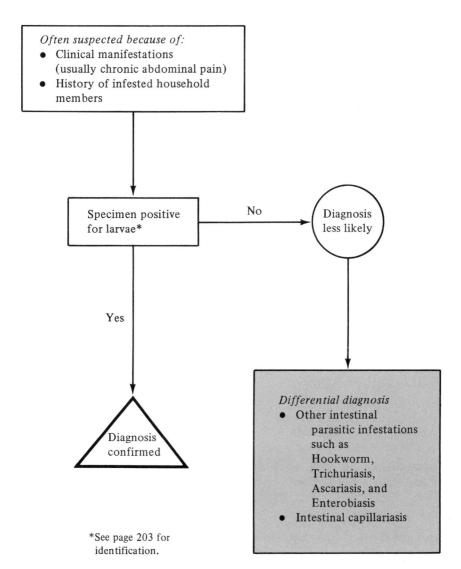

Often suspected because of:
- Clinical manifestations
  (usually chronic abdominal pain)
- History of infested household
  members

Specimen positive
for larvae*

No → Diagnosis
less likely

Yes

Diagnosis
confirmed

Differential diagnosis
- Other intestinal
  parasitic infestations
  such as
  Hookworm,
  Trichuriasis,
  Ascariasis, and
  Enterobiasis
- Intestinal capillariasis

*See page 203 for
identification.

▶ **CLINICAL MANIFESTATIONS**

1. Primary—single painless chancre and regional lymphadenopathy.
2. Secondary—symmetric mucocutaneous erythematous macular or papulo-squamous lesions (may occur on palms and soles), patchy alopecia, condylomata latum. Variable constitutional symptoms including fever, weight loss, malaise, and headache.
3. Latent—asymptomatic.
4. Tertiary—general paresis, tabes dorsalis, endarteritis, obliteration of vasa vasorum, iritis, gummas, aortic aneurysms.
5. Congenital—TORCHES' syndrome with rash, jaundice, hepatosplenomegaly, coryza, pneumonia, osteochondritis, and failure to thrive.

▶ **EPIDEMIOLOGY**

Agent: Spirochetal—*Treponema pallidum.*

Reservoir: Humans; especially homosexuals and prostitutes.

Transmission: By direct contact of primary lesions, by contact with body fluids, or secretions of patients in infectious primary and secondary stages, and by prenatal intrauterine infection.

Incubation period: 10 days to 3 weeks.

Period of communicability: Variable.

▶ **DIAGNOSTIC PROCEDURES**

Serology: Nonspecific—reagin antibody tests such as VDRL (flocculation), complement fixation (Kolmer's), or agglutination (RPR). *Specific*—treponemal antibody tests such as FTA-ABS (immunofluorescence), TPI (immobilization), or TPHA (hemagglutination).

Other: Dark-field examination of primary chancre or condylomata lata for *T. pallidum.*

▶ **MANAGEMENT**

Patient treatment: See chart on page 99.

Patient isolation: None required. Sexual contact discouraged until 24 hours after adequate treatment completed.

Management of contacts: Report, examine, and treat all sexual contacts of infected person.

Other: Educate public to have evaluations of suspected lesions, and to adequately report all known sexual contacts of infected individuals to local health authorities.

Often suspected because of:

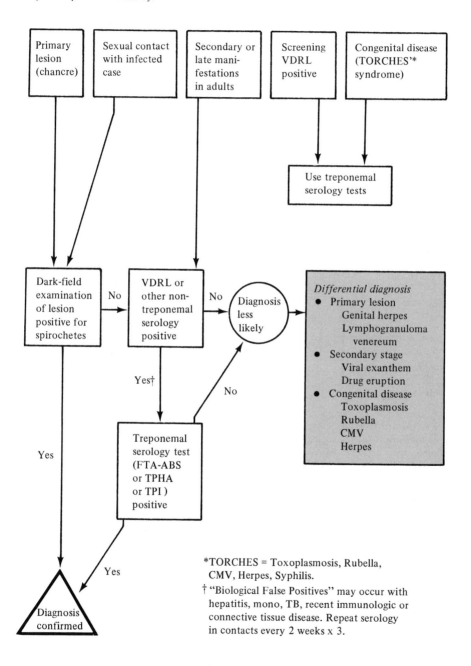

Primary lesion (chancre)

Sexual contact with infected case

Secondary or late manifestations in adults

Screening VDRL positive

Congenital disease (TORCHES'* syndrome)

Use treponemal serology tests

Dark-field examination of lesion positive for spirochetes

No

VDRL or other non-treponemal serology positive

No

Diagnosis less likely

Yes†

No

Yes

Treponemal serology test (FTA-ABS or TPHA or TPI) positive

Differential diagnosis
- Primary lesion
  Genital herpes
  Lymphogranuloma
    venereum
- Secondary stage
  Viral exanthem
  Drug eruption
- Congenital disease
  Toxoplasmosis
  Rubella
  CMV
  Herpes

Yes

Diagnosis confirmed

*TORCHES = Toxoplasmosis, Rubella, CMV, Herpes, Syphilis.

† "Biological False Positives" may occur with hepatitis, mono, TB, recent immunologic or connective tissue disease. Repeat serology in contacts every 2 weeks x 3.

RECOMMENDED THERAPY FOR SYPHILIS

Stage	Patients without penicillin allergy	Patients with penicillin allergy
Primary, secondary, or early latent (less than 1 year)	Benzathine penicillin G 2.4 million units IM single dose (1.2 million units in each buttock) *or* Aqueous procaine penicillin G, 600,000 units daily for 8 days	Erythromycin base, stearate, or ethyl succinate, 2 gm daily for 15 days *or* Tetracycline hydrochloride 2 gm daily for 15 days
Late latent or latent of uncertain duration	CSF normal—treat as primary CSF abnormal—treat as for neurosyphilis	Lumbar puncture CSF normal—treat as primary CSF abnormal—treat as neurosyphilis
Late neurosyphilis[a] **(asymptomatic or symptomatic)**	Aqueous procaine penicillin G, 600,000 units daily for 14 days *or* Aqueous penicillin G 12–24 million units/day IV for at least 10 days	Erythromycin base, stearate, or ethyl succinate 2 gm daily for 30 days *or* Tetracycline hydrochloride 2 gm daily for 30 days

RECOMMENDED THERAPY FOR SYPHILIS (Cont.)

Stage	Patients without penicillin allergy	Patients with penicillin allergy
Late cardiovascular or benign tertiary	Benzathine penicillin G 2.4 million units IM weekly for 3 weeks *or* Aqueous procaine penicillin G, 600,000 units weekly for 10 days	Treat as for neurosyphilis
Congenital (treat all neonates with either proved or suspected congenital syphilis)	Aqueous procaine penicillin G, 500,000 units/kg/day for at least 10 days *or* Aqueous penicillin G, 50,000 units/kg/day in two divided daily doses for at least 10 days *or* *Only if CSF normal—* benzathine penicillin G 50,000 units/kg in a single dose	Antibiotics other than penicillin should not be used

[a]Benzathine penicillin G has given inferior results for treatment of symptomatic neurosyphilis. Although only erythromycin or tetracycline was recommended by the CDC Syphilis Therapy Advisory Committee for CNS syphilis, chloramphenicol may be theoretically preferable, since it reaches higher concentrations in the CSF.

▶ **CLINICAL MANIFESTATIONS**

1. Pain or spasm of the muscles around a wound may be the first symptom, but stiffness usually starts in the jaw and neck. Rigidity may progress to include trunk and extremities within 24–48 hours.
2. Respiratory distress and death are common (greater than 50% fatality). Fever is a bad prognostic sign.

▶ **EPIDEMIOLOGY**

Agent: Bacterial—the tetanus bacillus (*Clostridium tetani,* toxin-producing).

Reservoir: Soil and the intestinal tract of animals, including humans.

Transmission: Spores from the bacteria enter the body through contaminated wounds, many of which are minor, or through the umbilicus of the newborn.

Incubation period: 3 days to 3 weeks, usually 7–10 days.

Period of communicability: None. Not transmitted person to person.

Duration of immunity: Unknown. Vaccination boosters recommended at least every 10 years, even after infection.

▶ **DIAGNOSTIC PROCEDURES**

Cultures: Specimen—material from wound (results often negative).
          Media—blood agar (anaerobic incubation).

Other: The spinal fluid is normal.

▶ **MANAGEMENT**

Patient treatment: Hospitalization in a quiet, dark room. Good respiratory supportive care. Control of spasms with sedatives such as diazepam or chlorpromazine. Human tetanus immune globulin 3000–6000 units IM *or* tetanus antitoxin 100,000 units IM (after horse serum sensitivity testing). Antibiotics such as penicillin or tetracycline for at least 10 days, and start immunizations.

Patient isolation: None.

Immunization: Tetanus toxoid. See immunization schedule, page 218).

Other: Careful cleaning and debridement of wounds is an important preventive measure. Booster immunization of women of childbearing age can prevent tetanus neonatorum.

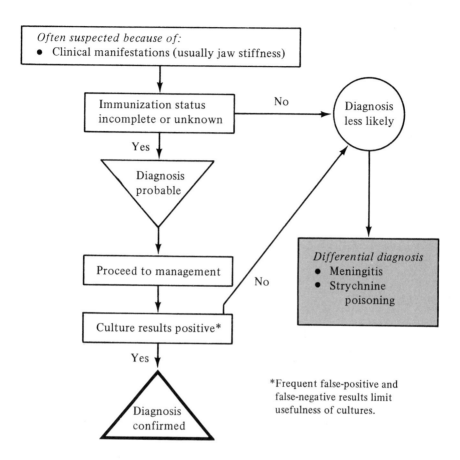

*Frequent false-positive and
false-negative results limit
usefulness of cultures.

GUIDE TO TETANUS PROPHYLAXIS IN WOUND MANAGEMENT

History of Tetanus Immunization (Doses)	Clean, Minor Wounds		All Other Wounds	
	Td[a]	TIG[b]	Td	TIG
Uncertain	Yes	No	Yes	Yes
0–1	Yes	No	Yes	Yes
2	Yes	No	Yes	No[c]
3 or more	No[d]	No	No[e]	No

[a]Td = Tetanus and diphtheria toxoids, adult type. In children 6 or under use DTP.
[b]TIG = Tetanus immune globulin. If unavailable, antitoxin may be used (3000–5000 units)
[c]Unless wound more than 24 hours old.
[d]Unless more than 10 years since last dose.
[e]Unless more than 5 years since last dose.

▶ CLINICAL MANIFESTATIONS

1. Vaginal discharge in females.
2. Asymptomatic in males.

▶ EPIDEMIOLOGY

Agent: Protozoan—*Trichomonas vaginalis.*

Reservoir: Humans.

Transmission: Direct (usually sexual) or indirect (contaminated article) contact.

Incubation period: 4–20 days.

Period of communicability: Duration of infection.

▶ DIAGNOSTIC PROCEDURES

Other: Direct microscopic examination.

▶ MANAGEMENT

Patient treatment: Vinegar and water douches often helpful. Metronidazole 2 gm PO once, 500 mg PO bid x 5 days or 250 mg PO tid x 10 days for both patient and sexual partner. Choose dosage and schedule considering side effects and compliance. *Note:* Avoid alcohol consumption during treatment with metronidazole.

Patient isolation: Avoid sexual intercourse until 10 days after onset of treatment.

Management of contacts: Treat sexual partners even if asymptomatic.

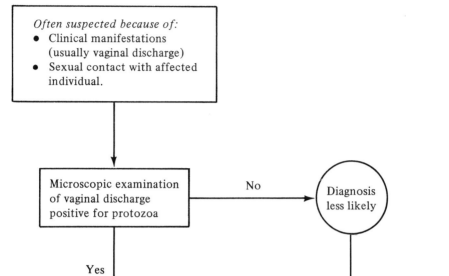

▶ **CLINICAL MANIFESTATIONS**

1. Usually asymptomatic.
2. Heavy infestation more commonly occurs in children and may cause abdominal pain, bloody diarrhea, and occasionally rectal prolapse.

▶ **EPIDEMIOLOGY**

Agent: Parasitic—*Trichuris trichiura,* a nematode.

Reservoir: Humans.

Transmission: By ingestion of soil contaminated with parasite eggs.

Incubation period: Indefinite.

Period of communicability: Not transmitted person to person, but ova may be found in stools for several years.

▶ **DIAGNOSTIC PROCEDURES**

Other: Microscopic examination of stool may demonstrate eggs within 90 days after initial infestation.

▶ **MANAGEMENT**

Patient treatment: Light infestations are usually asymptomatic, self-limited, and require no treatment. Mebendazole 100 mg PO, bid x 3 days is drug of choice for heavy infestations. Thiabendazole 25 mg/kg PO, bid x 3 days is an alternative but less effective drug.

Patient isolation: None.

Management of contacts: None, but other household members, especially children and playmates, frequently infested.

Other: Sanitary disposal of sewage.

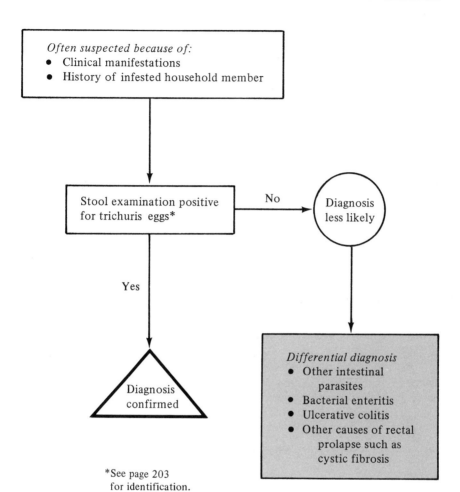

Often suspected because of:
- Clinical manifestations
- History of infested household member

Stool examination positive
for trichuris eggs*

No → Diagnosis less likely

Yes

Diagnosis confirmed

Differential diagnosis
- Other intestinal parasites
- Bacterial enteritis
- Ulcerative colitis
- Other causes of rectal prolapse such as cystic fibrosis

*See page 203 for identification.

▶ **CLINICAL MANIFESTATIONS**

1. Initial infections are usually asymptomatic, often become "inactive."
2. Pulmonary "active" infection may cause chronic or intermittent cough, fever, weight loss, and hemoptysis.
3. Extrapulmonary infections may develop in blood, meninges, lymph nodes, kidneys, skin, and other organs.

▶ **EPIDEMIOLOGY**

Agent: Bacterial—*Mycobacterium tuberculosis.*

Reservoir: Humans (bovine tuberculosis is transmitted to humans by unpasteurized dairy products).

Transmission: Usually by inhalation of infected sputum (droplet nuclei).

Incubation period: 2–10 weeks for primary lesions.

Period of communicability: As long as sputum, urine, or secretions positive.

▶ **DIAGNOSTIC PROCEDURES**

Cultures: Specimens—Usually sputum and tracheobronchial and gastric washings. Media—Lowenstein-Jensen in CO_2 environment.

Skin tests: Multiple puncture tests (e.g., tine) are good for screening. Confirm doubtful or positive reactions with Mantoux test (PPD), 5 tuberculin units (TU) in 0.1 ml of solution, injected intracutaneously. Measure induration in 48–72 hours: 0–4 mm = negative, 5–9 mm = doubtful (repeat in 1 month), and 10 mm or more = positive. *Note:* BCG history can cause 15 mm PPD reactions.

Other: Examine chest X ray for calcifications, apical lucencies, or coin lesion. Microscopic examination of specimens for acid-fast bacilli is useful.

▶ **MANAGEMENT**

Patient treatment

1. PPD positive without active disease—consider INH for 1 year. *Note:* Factors which *increase* the need for treatment: age under 30 (less chance of INH hepatitis), documented PPD conversion within 2 years, definite history of contact, ongoing exposure, concurrent illness (e.g., diabetes and lymphoma) and high-risk situations (e.g., partial gastrectomy and fibrocalcific pulmonary residuals).
2. Pulmonary, noncavity, active disease (sputum positive): INH and PAS or ethambutol for 18–25 months.
3. Other forms of active disease—INH, PAS and streptomycin for 2–4 months then INH and PAS for 2 years.
   Dosages—INH 10–30 mg/kg/day (300 mg max.) single dose, PO, IM, or IV. PAS 200 mg/kg/day (12 gm max.) in 3 doses, PO or IM. Streptomycin 20 mg/kg/day (1 gm max.) single dose IM.
   Alternatives for resistant organisms: ethionamide, ethambutol, rifampin.

(Continued on next page)

▶ MANAGEMENT (Cont.)

Patient isolation: Respiratory isolation (see page 232) until cultures and smears are negative.

Immunization: BCG offers variable protection, consider only in areas where TB is highly endemic.

Management of contacts: Treat household contacts of infectious cases with INH for 12 months. Check all close contacts with skin tests.

Other measures: Improvement of poor social conditions such as overcrowding is probably the single most effective measure. Skin testing and/or chest X rays are an important part of health maintenance examination.

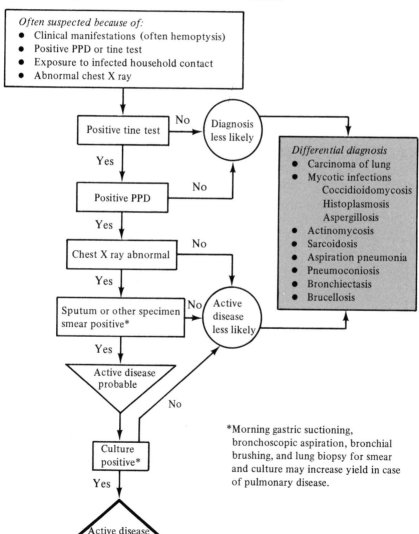

Often suspected because of:
- Clinical manifestations (often hemoptysis)
- Positive PPD or tine test
- Exposure to infected household contact
- Abnormal chest X ray

Positive tine test — No → Diagnosis less likely

Yes

Positive PPD — No → (Diagnosis less likely)

Yes

Chest X ray abnormal — No → Active disease less likely

Yes

Sputum or other specimen smear positive* — No → Active disease less likely

Yes

Active disease probable

No

Culture positive*

Yes

Active disease confirmed

Differential diagnosis
- Carcinoma of lung
- Mycotic infections
  - Coccidioidomycosis
  - Histoplasmosis
  - Aspergillosis
- Actinomycosis
- Sarcoidosis
- Aspiration pneumonia
- Pneumoconiosis
- Bronchiectasis
- Brucellosis

*Morning gastric suctioning, bronchoscopic aspiration, bronchial brushing, and lung biopsy for smear and culture may increase yield in case of pulmonary disease.

▶ **CLINICAL MANIFESTATIONS**

1. Variable symptoms including fever, headache, malaise, and constipation. Diarrhea, a mild rash, splenomegaly, and lymphadenopathy may also occur.
2. Fatality with treatment is less than 2%. *Note:* Paratyphoid fever is a slightly milder disease due to *Salmonella paratyphi.*

▶ **EPIDEMIOLOGY**

Agent: Bacterial—*Salmonella typhi.*

Reservoir: Humans.

Transmission: Oral ingestion of contaminated materials, particularly raw fruits and vegetables, oysters and other shellfish, milk, and water.

Incubation period: Usually 1–3 weeks.

Period of communicability: As long as salmonella are present in the stool or urine. May be as long as 3 months. Almost 5% of cases become chronic carriers.

▶ **DIAGNOSTIC PROCEDURES**

Cultures: Specimens—blood and bone marrow are often positive early in the disease, stool and urine usually not until 10 days after onset. Media—bismuth sulfite.

Serology: Agglutination reactions often positive within 10 days.

1. Typhoid H titer (flagella) are not specific and not useful clinically.
2. Typhoid O titers (cell wall) are affected by other salmonella infections and typhoid vaccine, but indicate probable typhoid fever if titers are over 1 : 100.

Other: Leukopenia of 3–4000 WBC/mm^3 is characteristic.

▶ **MANAGEMENT**

Patient treatment: Ampicillin or chloramphenicol depending on the antibiotic sensitivity of the organism. Long-term ampicillin may be effective for treatment of carriers.

Patient isolation: Enteric precautions (see page 233) until at least three consecutive daily negative stool cultures and urine cultures. Patient and carriers should be restricted from commercial food handling.

Immunization: Vaccine is of limited value but may be useful in:

1. Individuals planning to travel to endemic areas.
2. People living in the same house with a chronic carrier.
3. Groups exposed to ongoing outbreaks in which sanitary measures and education do not appear to control the epidemic.

Other: Water chlorination, adequate sewage disposal, and handwashing after toileting.

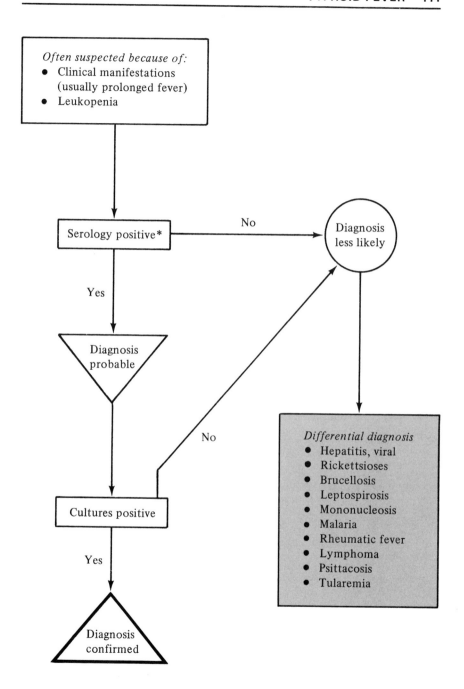

*False positives are common.

▶ CLINICAL MANIFESTATIONS

Varicella: (1) Acute onset with fever and fatigue. A skin eruption starts as an erythematous rash and progresses through maculopapular, vesicular, and crust stages. Lesions crust over in less than a week, and appear in crops over several days, mostly on the trunk and head. (2) Bacterial superinfection may occur. Varicella pneumonia and encephalomyelitis are uncommon complications.

Zoster (shingles): Dermatomal distribution of neuralgia, pruritus, and varicella lesions.

▶ EPIDEMIOLOGY

Agent: Viral—the varicella–zoster virus.

Reservoir: Humans.

Transmission: Direct contact, droplet spread, or indirect contact with articles contaminated by respiratory secretions or discharge from vesicles of infected person.

Incubation period: 2–3 weeks.

Period of communicability: From 5 days before the rash appears until all lesions crusted.

Duration of immunity: Usually lifelong. Infection may remain latent and re-occur years later as herpes zoster.

▶ DIAGNOSTIC PROCEDURES

Cultures: Specimens—vesicle fluid.
　　　　　Media—tissue culture.

Serology: Complement fixation titers and indirect immunofluorescent tests are useful. Obtain acute and convalescent sera.

Other: Scrapings of skin lesions can be examined microscopically for multi-nucleate giant epithelial cells (Giemsa stain).

▶ MANAGEMENT

Patient treatment: Symptomatic. Wet-to-dry compresses and oral antihistamines may help relieve itching. Bathing may help prevent superinfection.

Patient isolation: Keep home from school until all lesions crusted (about 6 days). If in hospital, strict or respiratory isolation (see page 232).

Management of contacts: Zoster immune globulin is advised for contacts with immunodeficiencies, particularly leukemia and Hodgkin's disease.

Other: Routine laundering of contaminated articles.

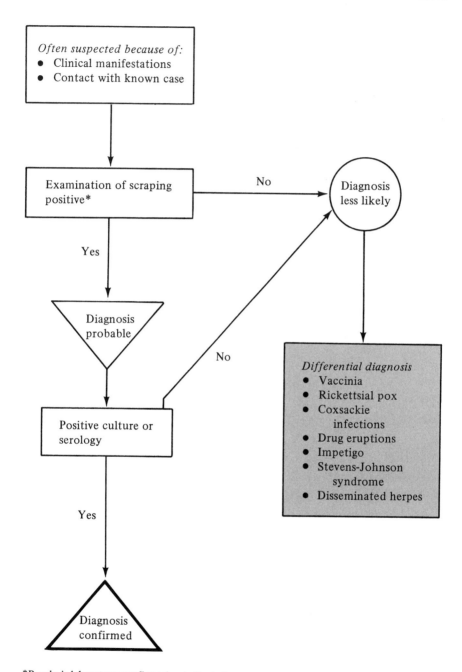

Often suspected because of:
- Clinical manifestations
- Contact with known case

Examination of scraping positive*

No → Diagnosis less likely

Yes

Diagnosis probable

No

Positive culture or serology

Differential diagnosis
- Vaccinia
- Rickettsial pox
- Coxsackie infections
- Drug eruptions
- Impetigo
- Stevens-Johnson syndrome
- Disseminated herpes

Yes

Diagnosis confirmed

*Rarely is laboratory confirmation indicated.

▶ **CLINICAL MANIFESTATIONS**

1. Commonly asymptomatic.
2. Sudden onset of fever, headache, backache, congestion, nausea, vomiting, jaundice, bradycardia, and hemorrhage (especially apistaxis and broccal bleeding).

▶ **EPIDEMIOLOGY**

Agent: Viral—an arbovirus.

Reservoir: Humans, mosquitos, and monkeys (in rural "endemic" yellow fever).

Transmission: By the bite of an infected mosquito.

Incubation period: 3–6 days.

Period of communicability: From several days before to up to 5 days after fever starts, the blood of man is infectious for mosquitos (which remain infected for life).

Duration of immunity: Lifelong.

▶ **DIAGNOSTIC PROCEDURES**

Culture: Specimen—blood, liver.
Media—tissue culture or suckling mice inoculation (in special laboratories only).

Serology: A fourfold rise in antibodies confirms the diagnosis.

Skin test: None.

Other: Liver biopsies may show characteristic necrosis and inclusion bodies.

▶ **MANAGEMENT**

Patient treatment: Supportive.

Patient isolation: For first 5 days of illness keep patient away from mosquitos by screening or spraying.

Immunization: A single subcutaneous or IM dose of the live, attenuated virus vaccine is recommended for those who will be exposed because of travel, residence, or occupation. Boosters should be given every 10 years. Vaccine grown in eggs.

Management of contacts: Immunize susceptible household and neighborhood members. Observe for symptoms.

Other: Mosquito surveillance and eradication.

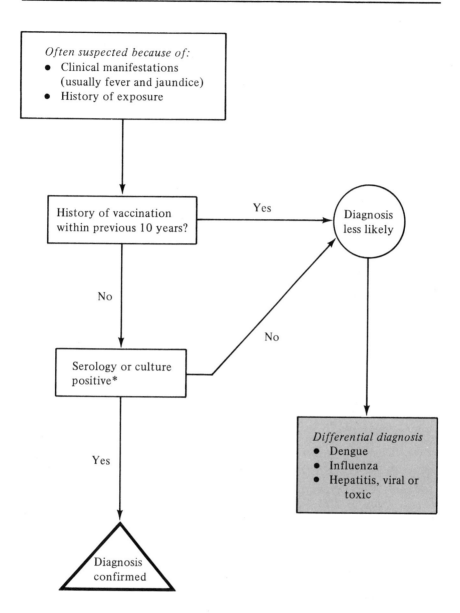

*Serology requires fourfold increase to confirm diagnosis.
Liver biopsy may be helpful for immediate presumptive
diagnosis.

Disease	Clinical Manifestations	Epidemiology				
		Agent	Reservoir	Transmission	Incubation Period	Period of Communicability
Anaerobic infections	Variable, including pneumonitis and abscesses, wound infections, bacteremia, meningitis, sinusitis, and omphalitis	Several hundred species of bacteroides, clostridium, streptococci, and other genera	Usually humans (normal flora)	During vaginal delivery, aspiration, surgical, or traumatic bowel spillage, and others	Usually from 1–5 days	While lesions are open
Anthrax	Skin— usually painless, black eschar, lymphadenopathy and septicemia Lungs— pneumonitis GI tract— abdominal distress	*Bacillus anthracis*	Contaminated soil or animal products	By direct contact with animal products (hides, etc.), inhalation of spores, eating contaminated meat	Less than 7 days	While lesions are active
E. coli infections	Variable. Common cause of UTIs, (for diarrhea due to enteropathogenic *E. coli,* see page 32)	*E. coli*	Usually human GI tract	Usually unknown	Unknown	Usually not transmitted person to person
Klebsiella infections	Variable, including pneumonia, cholecystitis, urinary tract infections, and sepsis	*Klebsiella pneumoniae*	Usually from GI tract or hospital environment	Usually unknown or in hospital	Variable	Usually not transmitted person to person
Legionnaires' disease	Pneumonia, often with GI and CNS symptoms	*Legionella pneumophila,* 4 serogroups	Unknown; possibly air cooling units	Probably air-borne	Unknown; possibly one to ten days	Unknown
Listeria infections	Neonatal sepsis, meningitis, and abscesses. Usually asymptomatic or mild infection in adults	*Listeria monocytogenes*	Probably human	Usually unknown transplacental, or during vaginal delivery	Unknown	Unknown
Proteus infections	Variable, including upper UTIs, kidney stones, pneumonia, and sepsis	*Proteus mirabilis* or *vulgaris*	Usually human GI tract	Usually unknown or by urinary tract manipulation	Variable	Usually not transmitted person to person

	Diagnostic Procedures			Management			
	Cultures		Other	Patient	Patient	Immuni-	Other Preventive
Specimen	Media		Tests*	Treatment	Isolation	zation	Measures
Depends on site	Transport and culture anaerobically	None		Usually ampicillin, penicillin, or carbeni-cillin (except B. fragilis) or chloram-phenicol or clindamycin	Wound isolation precautions	None	Aseptic surgical technique
Pulmonary or lesion discharges, blood	Special media, animal inoculation		Gram stain microscopic examination of smears for organisms. FA techniques are useful	Penicillin, erythro-mycin, tetracycline, or chloram-phenicol	Strict isolation	For high-risk veter-inarians and others (contact CDC)	Control of animal disease and restriction on importation of possibly con-taminated animal products
Depends on site	Mueller-Hinton or blood agar	None		Usually sensitive to ampicillin, cephalo-sporins, sul-fonamides, tetracycline, and others	Usually none	None	None
Depends on site	Mueller-Hinton or blood agar	Gram stain of smear may be helpful but not diagnostic		Usually cephalo-sporins and/ or aminogly-cosides (except gentamicin)	For hospital-ized patients with multiple-resistant organisms depending on site	None	None
Pleural fluid (hard to culture)	Mueller-Hinton with 2% Isovitalex			Erythro-mycin	None	None	None
Blood, CF, meconium, or others		On gram stain, similarity to diphtheroids may be misleading		Usually ampicillin and/or kanamycin or gentamicin	Mainly to protect other hospitalized infants	None	None
Depends on site	Mueller-Hinton or blood agar	None		Ampicillin or a cepha-losporin. P. vulgaris may require an aminoglyco-side (except kanamycin)	Usually none	None	Sterile technique for urinary tract manipulation

*No serology or skin tests are available for bacterial infections except for anthrax (indirect hemagglutination titers) and Legionnaires' disease (indirect fluorescent antibody titers).

MISCELLANEOUS CHLAMYDIAL INFECTIONS

| Disease | Most Common Clinical Manifestations | Epidemiology | | | | |
		Agent	Reservoir	Transmission	Incubation Period	Period of Communicability
Lymphogranuloma venereum	Inguinal lymphadenopathy and bubos	A chlamydia	Humans	Usually sexual	5–21 days	While lesions are present (weeks to months)
Nongonococcal urethritis (NGU), Pelvic inflammatory disease (PID), and vaginitis other than IGC, trichomoniasis, or candidiasis	Dysuria, urethral discharge	Usually C. trachomatis	Humans	Usually sexual	Unknown	Unknown
Neonatal inclusion conjunctivitis (inclusion blenorrhea)	Conjunctivitis	C. trachomatis	Humans	By contact with mother's genital tract during delivery	2–15 days	Unknown
Trachoma conjunctivitis (non-neonatal)	Conjunctivitis	C. trachomatis	Humans	Eye to eye via articles, fingers, and insects	5–14 days	During acute illness
Infant pneumonia	Cough, fever, and other symptoms of pneumonitis	C. trachomatis	Humans	Unknown, may follow latent newborn infection	Unknown	During acute illness
Psittacosis (ornithosis)	Usually mild with fever, headache, anorexia, productive cough, and other symptoms of pneumonitis	C. psittaci	Birds	Contact with birds and their environment	4–15 days	During acute illness

	MISCELLANEOUS CHLAMYDIAL INFECTIONS (Cont.)					
Diagnostic Procedures			**Management**			
Cultures			*Patient Treatment*	*Patient Isolation*	*Immuni- zation*	*Other Preventive Measures*
Specimens	*Media*	*Serology[a]*				
Pus from bubo	Tissue cultures, animal inocu- lation	CF	Sulfona- mides or tetracycline x 21 days	None	None	Wear gloves when examining genital lesions
Urethral or vaginal swab	Tissue cultures, animal inocu- lation	CF	Sulfona- mides or tetracycline x 2-3 weeks	None	None	No intercourse during treatment
Conjunc- tival discharge or scrapings	Tissue cultures, animal inocu- lation	CF[b]	Ophthalmic ointment or solution (sulfa or tetracycline) qid x 2 weeks	None	None	None
Conjunc- tival discharge or scrapings	Tissue cultures, animal inocu- lation	CF and several other tests are useful[b]	Sulfona- mides or tetracycline PO x 3 weeks, *plus* ophthalmic ointment or solution x 6 weeks	None	None	Limit sharing of towels, etc.; handwashing may help
Pulmonary secretions	Tissue cultures, animal inocu- lations	CF	Sulfona- mides	Respiratory precautions to protect other infants	None	None
Processing cultures is dangerous and not recommended		CF	Tetracyclines PO until at least 10 days past febrile stage	Respiratory precautions x 2 weeks	None	Educate bird handlers

[a] No skin tests are applicable to chlamydial infections.
[b] Other diagnostic procedures for neonatal conjunctivitis and trachoma conjunctivitis: Giemsa stain reveals cytoplasmic inclusion bodies in epithelial cells.

FOOD-BORNE DISEASES*

Agent	Clinical Manifestations
S. aureus (toxin)	Abrupt onset of nausea, vomiting, cramps, diarrhea, and prostration
C. perfringens	Nausea, diarrhea, cramps
C. botulinum (toxin)	Vomiting, diarrhea, diplopia, dry mouth, weakness, sore throat, and respiratory paralysis
B. cereus	Vomiting, cramps and/or diarrhea
E. coli (toxin)	Cramps, watery diarrhea, prostration, occasional fever
Salmonellae	Persistent diarrhea, nausea, vomiting, fever
Shigellae	Cramps, persistent, often bloody diarrhea, fever
Streptococcus, group A	Sore throat, nausea, vomiting, fever
Vibrio parahemolyticus	Cramps, watery diarrhea, often nausea, vomiting, headache, fever
Mushrooms	Depends upon type of mushroom; may be mental; GI myalgia or late hepatorenal failure
Metals and chemicals, red-tide shellfish toxin	GI symptoms commonest; also neurological, cyanosis, metallic taste
Parasites	GI, hepatic
Hepatitis A	Fever, jaundice, GI
Brucellosis	Insidious, fever, weakness, myalgias
Carbon monoxide	Often presents as "food poisoning"

*Cultures of food, vomitus, feces, and toxin levels in food, serum, and stool may be useful. Not transmitted person-to-person, no isolation or contact management required. Enteric precautions for food handlers. 50% of bacterial food poisoning caused by *Staphylococcus aureus* and *Clostridium perfringens*.

FOOD-BORNE DISEASES (Cont.)

Incubation	Usual Sources
1–8 hours	Meats, ham, dairy products, custards, pastries— contaminated by human nasal discharge or skin lesions
8–24 hours	Meats, (beef, turkey, chicken) in stews, gravies— contaminated by human feces or soil
12–36 hours	Home-canned vegetables and fruits and fish— contaminated by feces or soil
1–16 hours	Custards, and sources contaminated by soil
6–36 hours	Contaminated water
6–48 hours	Poultry, meat, dairy products—associated with pets
7–168 hours	Food and water
24–72 hours	Dairy products, meat
4–96 hours	Fish and shellfish
1/2–48 hours	Mushrooms
3 minutes–3 hours	Seasonings (sodium glutamate), pesticide, nitrate, CN, heavy metals, etc., or histamine
Days–weeks	Raw or undercooked meats
15–60 days	Shellfish, milk, water, other food contaminated by urine or feces
5–21 days	Raw milk or cheese
Minutes–hours	Air

Adapted from Eisenberg, M., et al., *Manual of Antimicrobial Therapy and Communicable Diseases 1976,* State of Washington, Department of Social and Health Services.

MISCELLANEOUS FUNGAL INFECTIONS

Disease	Clinical Manifestations	Agent	Reservoir	Transmission	Incubation Period	Period of Communicability
				Epidemiology		
Aspergillosis	Localized disseminated or granulomatous lesions. May involve any organ, primarily in immunosuppressed patients	Usually *Aspergillus fumigatus*	A ubiquitous fungus	By inhalation of spores	Unknown, days to weeks	Not transmitted person to person
Blastomycosis	Granulomatous formations of skin and other organs	*Blastomyces dermatitidis* or *brasiliensis*	Unknown, probably soil	Unknown, probably by inhalation of spores	Unknown	Unknown
Coccidioidomycosis	Often asymptomatic; variable from rash and influenza-like syndrome to granulomatous formations of skin, lung, and other organs	*Coccidioides immitis*	Spore-contaminated soil in arid parts of southwest US, Mexico, Argentina	By inhalation of spores in dust, or pus inoculated into skin	1–3 weeks	Usually not transmitted person to person
Cryptococcosis (torulosis)	Often asymptomatic; variable from minor respiratory infection to granulomatous lesions of any organs	*Cryptococcus neoformans*	Pigeon excreta fertilized soil; world-wide	By inhalations of yeasts in dust	Unknown	Not transmitted person to person

MISCELLANEOUS FUNGAL INFECTIONS (Cont.)						
Diagnostic Procedures					*Management**	
Cultures			*Skin*		*Patient*	*Other Preventive*
Specimens	*Media*	*Serology*	*Tests*	*Other*	*Treatment*	*Measures*
Depends on site of infection	Sabouraud or brain-heart infusion	Precipitin tests are not confirma-tory	May be useful	Biopsies useful	Ampho-tericin B	None
Depends on site of infection	Sabouraud or brain-heart infusion (*B. brasiliensis* also grows on blood agar)	CF titers not con-firmatory	Not reliable	KOH prep of sputum, etc., may show budding yeast	Ampho-tericin B	None
[Culturing may be hazardous. Consult with health department.]		CF titers rise in several months, $\geq 1:32$ suggests dissemina-tion. Precipitin and other tests also useful	Helpful, positive in 3–6 weeks, but may be negative in severe disease (testing alters serology)	Soil cultures may reveal fungus	Ampho-tericin B	Disinfect secretion-contaminated articles. Dust control in endemic areas
Depends on site of infection	Sabouraud	Various agglutina-tion and fluorescent antibody tests available	Not reliable	Wet india ink mounts of specimens may reveal encapsulated yeasts	Ampho-tericin B for severe infections only	None

*Not transmitted person to person. No patient isolation, contact management or immunization required.

MISCELLANEOUS PARASITIC INFESTATIONS

Disease	Most Common Clinical Manifestations	Epidemiology				
		Agent	Reservoir	Transmission	Incubation Period	Period of Communicability
Balantidiasis	Diarrhea	*Balantidium coli*	Humans and swine	Fecal-oral, contaminated food	Variable	Duration of infestation
Trypanosomiasis, American (Chagas' disease)	Fever, malaise, lymphadenopathy, palpebral edema	*Trypanosoma cruzi*	Humans and other animals	Reduviid bug bites, transfusions, transplacental	5–15 days	Unknown
Larva migrans, cutaneous (creeping eruption)	Skin eruption, itching	Ancylostoma spp	Cats and dogs	Penetration of contaminated skin by larvae	1–3 days	Not transmitted person to person
Larva migrans, visceral (toxocariasis)	Pulmonary irritation with wheezing	*T. canis* and *cati*	Dogs and cats	By eating contaminated soil	1 week	Not transmitted person to person
Tapeworm infestations	Intestinal irritation; liver, lung, brain, or other mass lesions (cysticercosis by *T. solium*)	Taenia spp, *saginata* (beef) *solium* (pork) *latum* (fish)	Humans and intermediate hosts	By eating contaminated meat; fecal-oral route for *T. solium* only	Variable, depends on agent, may be years	Unknown; only *T. solium* transmitted person to person
Hydatid cyst disease	Liver, lung, brain, or other mass lesions (hydatid cysts)	*Echinococcus granulosus* and *multilocularis*	Dogs, wolves, foxes	By ingesting eggs from animal feces	Variable, may be years	Not transmitted person to person
Toxoplasmosis	Lymphadenopathy, infectious mono syndrome, chorioretinitis; congenital infections may cause jaundice, rash, seizures, microcephaly, (TORCHES' syndrome)	*Toxoplasma gondii*, a protozoan	Humans and other animals, cats are intermediate hosts	By ingesting soil, sand, food; by transfusions; transplacental	Variable, may be months	Unknown, only person-to-person transmission is parenteral

	MISCELLANEOUS PARASITIC INFESTATIONS (Cont.)					
Diagnostic Procedures					Management[a]	
	Cultures		Skin		Patient	Preventive
Specimens	Media	Serology	Tests	Other	Treatment	Measures
None	None	None	None	Micro exam of feces for cysts and trophozoites	Tetracycline	Sanitary disposal of feces
Blood	Special media	Yes	None	Direct blood smear	None; nitrofuran[b] primaquine[b]	Bed nets
None	None	None	None	Micro-identification of larvae from skin	Thiabenda-zole	Deworming of animals; control of stray animals and contaminated beaches
None	None	CF and precipitin tests for cysticer-cosis are useful	None	Micro exam of human feces for proglottids or eggs	Niclosamide; surgical removal of mass lesion	Proper cooking of meat, proper animal slaughter and meat inspection
None	None	None	None	Eosinophilia; elevated iso-agglutinins	Thiaben-dazole steroids[b,c]	Proper meat handling
None	None	CF, HA and others are useful	Yes, useful	None	Surgical	Proper food handling
Blood, CSF, saliva, biopsy specimens	Animal inoculation	CF, FA, and others are useful	Yes, useful	Micro exam of smears and tissues with Giemsa, PAS, and H & E stains	Sulfadiazine *plus* pyri-methamine[b]	Proper cooking of all meats, covering of sand boxes

[a] No immunization; patient isolation not required except as noted for Larva migrans, visceral, and Filiariasis.
[b] Benefits not well proven.
[c] Patient isolation for those with *T. solium* only.

(Continued on next page)

MISCELLANEOUS PARASITIC INFESTATIONS (Cont.)

Disease	Most Common Clinical Manifestations	Agent	Epidemiology			
			Reservoir	Transmission	Incubation Period	Period of Communicability
Trichinosis	Gastroenteritis, muscle aches, generalized inflammation of many organs	*Trichinella spiralis*	Swine, bear, and other mammals	By eating infected meat, especially pork	2–28 days	Not transmitted person to person
Filiariasis	Variable, ranging from fever and lymphadenitis to elephantiasis	*Wuchereria bancrofti* and other filarial worms	Humans	By mosquito bites	Usually several months	Not transmitted directly person to person
Leish-maniasis, cutaneous	Ulcerating or nodular skin and/or mucous membrane lesions	*Leishmania brasiliensis* or *mexicana,* a protozoa	Humans and other mammals	By the bite of phlebo-tomus sand flies	From days to months	Usually not transmitted person to person
Leish-maniasis, visceral	Fever, hepato-splenomegaly, anemia; often fatal if untreated	*L. donovarvi*	Humans and other mammals	By the bite of phlebo-tomus sand flies	Usually 2–4 months, up to several years	Not transmitted person to person

			MISCELLANEOUS PARASITIC INFESTATIONS (Cont.)			
		Diagnostic Procedures			*Management[a]*	
	Cultures		*Skin*		*Patient*	*Preventive*
Specimens	*Media*	*Serology*	*Tests*	*Other*	*Treatment*	*Measures*
None	None	CF, precipitin, and others are useful	Yes, useful	Micro exam of muscle biopsy; eosinophilia	Thiabenda-zole[b]	Proper cooking of meat
None	None	CF and other titers of limited utility	Not reliable	Microfilariae on blood films	Diethyl-carbama-zine[c]	Control of vectors
Material from lesions	Novy's and other special media	CF and other titers of limited utility	Not reliable	Micro exam of stained specimens for leishman-Donovan bodies	Antimony sodium gluconate and others	Control of local vectors and hosts
Blood and other specimens depending on site	Novy's and other special media	CF and other titers of limited utility	Not reliable	Micro exam of stained specimens for leishman-Donovan bodies	Antimony sodium gluconate and others	Control of local vectors and hosts

[a]No immunization; patient isolation not required except as noted for Larva migrans, visceral, and Filariasis.
[b]Benefits not well proven.
[c]Mosquito netting and repellent if practical in management.

MISCELLANEOUS RICKETTSIAL INFECTIONS

Disease	Most Common Clinical Manifestations	Epidemiology			
		Agent	Reservoir	Transmission	Incubation Period
Rocky Mountain spotted fever	Fever, headaches, myalgias, with macular and peteochial rash	*Rickettsia rickettsii*	Mammals; wood, dog, and rabbit ticks are vectors	By vector; ticks	3–12 days
Rickettsial pox	Local eschar and adenopathy, then malaise and vesicular rash	*R. akari*	Mice; mouse mites are vectors	By vector; mites	About 1 week
Epidemic typhus	Fever, chills, macular rash, and prostration	*R. prowazekii*	Humans; head and body lice are vectors	By vector; lice	1–2 weeks
Murine typhus	Fever, chills, macular rash, and prostration	*R. typhi*	Rats; fleas, and lice are vectors	By vector; fleas and lice	1–2 weeks
Q. fever (Query fever)	Often asymptomatic, or with fever, chills, headache, and pneumonia	*R. burnetii*	Domestic animals, like cattle	Usually airborne or by ingestion of contaminated animal products, (milk, etc.)	2–3 weeks

| MISCELLANEOUS RICKETTSIAL INFECTIONS (Cont.) | | | |
| Diagnostic Procedures[a] | Management[b] | | |
Serology	Patient Treatment	Immunization	Other Preventive Measures
CF, Weil-Felix[c]	Chloramphenicol or tetracycline	None recommended	Tick removal
CF	Chloramphenicol or tetracycline	None	Rodent control
CF, Weil-Felix[c]	Chloramphenicol or tetracycline	Military, laboratory, and other high-risk personnel (check with health department)	Insecticide (1% lindane)
CF, Weil-Felix[c]	Chloramphenicol or tetracycline	None	Insecticide applied to rat dwellings; rodent control
CF	Chloramphenicol or tetracycline	None recommended	Pasteurization

[a]No cultures or skin tests available or useful for rickettsial infections.
[b]No patient isolation required, since not transmitted person to person.
[c]False positives occur following proteus infections.

MISCELLANEOUS VIRAL INFECTIONS

Disease	Most Common Clinical Manifestations	Epidemiology				
		Agent	Reservoir	Transmission	Incubation Period	Period of Communicability
Arboviral en-cephalitides (California, Eastern equine, St. Louis, Venezuelan, Western equine)	Usually encephalitis and/or meningitis	Various viruses	Birds and mammals; humans are "dead-end" hosts	By mosquito bites	2–21 days depending on the virus	Probably not transmitted person to person
Cytomegalo-virus infections	Usually asymp-tomatic Congenital—failure to thrive, jaundice, rash, deafness, retardation (TORCHES' syndrome) Acquired—mono-like syndrome	CMV (herpes virus family)	Humans	Trans-placental, at time of birth, parenterally, sexually, and possibly by other means	Unknown	Unknown; perhaps several years
Entero-viral infections	Variable, (depends on virus) including fever, maculopapular rash, herpangina, pharyngitis, hand, foot and mouth disease, meningitis, paralysis, myocarditis, and enteritis	Coxsackie viruses (Groups A and B) and echo viruses	Humans	By direct contact via the fecal-oral or oro-oral route	2–14 days, but usually 3–5 days	Unknown; perhaps 2 weeks or longer
Erythema infectiosum (fifth disease)	Malar erythema followed by reticulated, maculopapular rash; usually seen in those 4–15 years of age	Probably a virus	Probably humans	Unknown	About 1–2 weeks	Unknown

MISCELLANEOUS VIRAL INFECTIONS (Cont.)						
Diagnostic Procedures[a]				Management[b]		
Cultures				Patient Treatment	Patient Isolation	Other Preventive Measures
Specimens	Media	Serology	Other			
Blood, brain	Tissue culture	HI, CF and others are useful; obtain paired sera	None	Supportive	None, but consider respiratory isolation for 2–4 days for those with VEE (virus in pharynx)	Vector control; immunization of horses
Urine, pharynx, cervix, blood, biopsy or autopsy material	Tissue culture	CF and HA tests are of limited diagnostic value; CMV-specific IgM antibodies in cord or infant serum are diagnostic of congenital infection	H and E, or Giemsa staining may reveal characteristic intranuclear inclusions	Adenine arabinoside is under investigation for use in congenital infections	Not practical, since most cases are undetected; consider isolation of infants	Personnel caring for known infected infant should wash hands carefully
Feces, throat, CSF	Tissue culture, animal inoculation	CF and neutralizing antibody titers help confirm infection but are only feasible if the virus is isolated	None	Supportive	Enteric precautions	None
None	None	None	None	Supportive	None	None

[a]No skin tests available for these viral infections.
[b]No immunization required (but see note for smallpox).

(Continued on next page)

			MISCELLANEOUS VIRAL INFECTIONS (Cont.)			
				Epidemiology		
Disease	*Most Common Clinical Manifestations*	*Agent*	*Reservoir*	*Transmission*	*Incubation Period*	*Period of Communicability*
Roseola infantum (exanthem subitum)	Several days of high fever followed by diffuse, maculopapular rash after fever breaks; limited to those 6 months to 4 years of age	Probably a virus	Probably humans	Unknown	About 10 days	Unknown
Smallpox (variola)	Fever and malaise followed in several days by a centrifugally distributed rash progressing from papules to pustules to scabs	Variola virus	Humans, up to 1978, when the last human case was reported in England. World-wide eradication has probably been ac-complished	Usually by close contact with patient or con-taminated articles	7–17 days	From appearance of rash until shedding of crusts (about 3 weeks)

MISCELLANEOUS VIRAL INFECTIONS (Cont.)						
Diagnostic Procedures[a]				Management[b]		
Cultures						Other
Specimens	Media	Serology	Other	Patient Treatment	Patient Isolation	Preventive Measures
None	None	None	None	Supportive	None	None
Blood, skin lesions, secretions, and crusts	Fertile chicken eggs	HI titers usually positive in 4–5 days; CF and precipitin tests also useful	Electron microscopy may reveal poxvirus in crust scrapings	Supportive[c]	Strict isolation	International reporting of suspect cases is critical

[a]No skin tests available for these viral infections.
[b]No immunization required (but see note for smallpox).
[c]Active immunization occasionally required for international travel.

		Epidemiology			
Disease Agents	*Usual Clinical Manifestations*	*Reservoir*	*Transmission*	*Incubation Period*	*Period of Communicability*
Adenoviruses	Variable, including pharyngitis, cough, fever, keratoconjunctivitis, and pneumonia	Humans	Direct contact and droplet spread	About 1 week	Usually several days, variable
Mycoplasma pneumoniae	Pharyngitis, tracheobronchitis, and/or pneumonia (diffuse or isolated infiltrates)	Humans	Direct contact and droplet spread	1–3 weeks	Unknown
Parainfluenza viruses	Rhinitis, bronchiolitis, pharyngitis, croup	Humans	Direct contact and droplet spread	2–7 days	Unknown, perhaps 1 week
Respiratory syncytial viruses	Bronchiolitis and/or pneumonia, particularly in young children	Humans	Direct contact and droplet spread	2–7 days	Unknown, perhaps 1 week
Rhinoviruses	The common cold	Humans	Direct contact and droplet spread	Several days	Unknown, perhaps several weeks

MISCELLANEOUS VIRAL RESPIRATORY INFECTIONS

MISCELLANEOUS VIRAL RESPIRATORY INFECTIONS (Cont.)				
Diagnostic Procedures[a,b]			Management[c]	
Cultures			Patient	Patient
Specimens	Media	Serology	Treatment	Isolation
Oropharyngeal swabbings	Tissue cultures	CF or neutralizing antibodies	None	Respiratory precautions in hospitals to protect high-risk pulmonary patients
Respiratory secretions, including sputum	Special media	CF, FA, and other titers are useful[d]	Erythromycin for at least 1 week	Respiratory precautions in hospitals to protect high-risk pulmonary patients
Oropharyngeal swabbings	Tissue culture	CF or neutralizing antibodies	None	Respiratory precautions in hospitals to protect high-risk pulmonary patients
Oropharyngeal swabbings	Tissue culture	CF or neutralizing antibodies	None	Respiratory precautions in hospitals to protect high-risk pulmonary patients
Isolation and serology tedious and *not* clinically practical			None	Respiratory precautions in hospitals to protect high-risk pulmonary patients

[a] Rarely warranted.
[b] No skin tests for viral respiratory infections
[c] No immunization for these infections.
[d] A fourfold rise in cold hemoglutinins (or single titer of $\geq 1 : 64$) is seen in more than 50% of patients.

3

ANTIMICROBIAL AGENTS

ANTIBIOTICS

▶ **AMOXICILLIN**

Usage

Same as ampicillin, but not useful in shigellosis.

Dosage

Pediatric: 20–40 mg/kg/day given in 3 doses PO.
Adult: 1-2 gm/day given in 3 doses PO.

How supplied

Capsules: 250 or 500 mg.
Liquid: 125 or 250 mg/5 cc.

Adverse reaction

Maculopapular rash common, especially in patients with infectious mononucleosis.

Notes

Produces less diarrhea and skin eruptions than ampicillin and is better absorbed, but usually more expensive.

▶ **AMPICILLIN**

Usage

A drug of first choice for most *Haemophilus influenzae,* shigella, salmonella, *E. coli,* enterococcus (*Streptococcus fecalis*).
Not active against penicillinase-producing organisms.

Dosage

Newborn: Under 1 week, 50–100 mg/kg/day in 2 doses IV or IM.
         1 week to 1 month, 75–225 mg/kg/day in 2 doses IV or IM.
Pediatric: 75–300 mg/kg/day in 4 doses PO, IV, or IM.
Adult: 2–12 gm/day in 4 doses PO, IV, or IM.

How supplied

Capsules: 250 or 500 mg.
Liquid: 125 mg/cc (usually in 100- or 200-cc bottles) or 250 mg/5 cc.

Adverse reactions

Maculopapular rash common, especially in patients with mononucleosis.

Drug interaction

Allopurinol—may cause skin rash.

▶ **AMPICILLIN (Cont.)**

Notes

Administer on empty stomach.

▶ **CARBENICILLIN**

Usage

A drug of choice for pseudomonas infections when used with gentamicin or tobramycin.

Dosage

Newborn: If under 1 week and low birth weight (under 2000 gm) 200 mg/kg/day in 3 doses IV or IM.
Pediatric: 400–600 mg/kg/day in 4–6 doses IV (PO and IM rarely indicated).
Adult: 500 mg/kg/day in 4–6 doses PO, IV, or IM. (2–6 gm/day IV or PO for susceptible UTIs).

How supplied

Tablets: 382 mg (in each 500 mg tablet of indanyl sodium salt).
Ampoules: 1, 2, or 5 gm.

Adverse reactions

Klebsiella or candida superinfections are common. Hypernatremia, hypokalemia, and rarely altered platelet function.

Drug interactions

Sometimes synergistic with gentamicin and tobramycin or amikacin in treatment of pseudomonal infection but physically incompatible in same IV bottle.

Notes

Each gram contains 4.7 mEq of sodium.
Limit PO use to urinary tract infection when other drugs are not effective, since resistant strains of pseudomonas may occur.

▶ **CEFAZOLIN**

Usage

See Cephalothin.

Dosage

Pediatric: 25–100 mg/kg/day in 3 or 4 doses IM or IV.
Adult: 1–6 gm/day in 2 doses IM or IV.

▶ **CEFAZOLIN (Cont.)**

How supplied

Ampoules: 250 and 500 mg/10 cc in 1, 5, and 10 gm vials.

Adverse reactions

See Cephalothin.

Notes

Better tolerated IM than is cephalothin. Risk of thrombosis less than cephalothin. Renal damage less than cephaloridine.

▶ **CEPHALOTHIN**

Usage

A drug of choice for most klebsiella infections. May also be useful for *S. aureus,* streptococcal, pneumococcal, *E. coli,* and *P. mirabilis* infections.

Dosage

Pediatric: 50–200 mg/kg/day in 4–6 doses IV or IM.
Adult: 4–12 gm/day in 6 doses IV or IM.

How supplied

Ampoules: 1, 2, 4, and 20 gm vials in various concentrations.

Adverse reactions

Painful IM and thrombophlebitis from IV infusion.
Probable cross allergenicity of penicillin and cephalosporins.
Rarely causes blood dyscrasias, hemolytic anemia, or renal toxicity.
Superinfection may occur upon prolonged therapy.

Notes

Cephapirin, cephradine, and cephaloridine are essentially equivalent drugs, but check dosages.
CSF levels: Poor; not recommended in cases of meningitis.

▶ **CEPHALEXIN**

Usage

See Cephalothin; usually reserved for treatment of less serious infections.

Dosage

Pediatric: 25–100 mg/kg/day in 4 doses PO.
Adult: 2–4 gm/day in 4 doses PO.

▶ **CEPHALEXIN (Cont.)**

How supplied

Capsules: 250 and 500 mg.
Liquid: 125 mg or 250 mg/5 cc.
Drops: 100 mg/cc.

Adverse reactions

Diarrhea and gastrointestinal distress may occur.

Notes

Cephradine is equivalent drug.
See Cephalothin for adverse effects.
Acid stable, may be given with meals.

▶ **CHLORAMPHENICOL**

Usage

A drug of choice for most *Salmonella typhi* and *Bacteroides fragilis* infections.
May also be useful for klebsiella, shigella, serratia, rickettsia, cholera, clostridia
infections, ampicillin resistant hemophilus infections, and most anaerobic
bacteria.
Limit use to severe infections.
Very useful in treatment of meningitis and brain abscess.

Dosage

Newborn: Under 1 week, 25 mg/kg/day single dose IV.
            1 week to 1 month, 50 mg/kg/day in 2 doses IV.
Pediatric: 50–100 mg/kg/day in 4 doses PO or IV.
Adult: 2–4 gm/day in 4 doses PO or IV.

How supplied

Capsules: 50, 100, and 250 mg.
Liquid: 125 mg/5 cc (palmitate).
Ampoule: 1 gm/10 cc (sodium succinate).
Also available in ophthalmic preparations and topical ointments.

Adverse reactions

Dose-related bone marrow depression may occur, so white count and platelets
should be monitored.
Aplastic anemia rare.
Gray-baby syndrome may occur if too high a dose given to neonates (monitoring
blood levels may be useful).

▶ **CHLORAMPHENICOL (Cont.)**

Drug interactions

By inhibiting breakdown of other drugs.
Tolbutamide: May cause hypoglycemia.
Anticoagulants: May increase anticoagulation.
Dilantin: May increase dilantin toxicity.
Bilirubin: May increase kernicterus in newborns.

Notes

CSF levels: Excellent.

▶ **CLINDAMYCIN**

Usage

A drug of choice for most *B. fragilis* infections, and active against most other anaerobes.
Limit use to serious anaerobic infections.

Dosage

Pediatric: 8–20 mg/kg/day in 4 doses PO, IV, or IM.
Adult: 1–3 gm/day in 4 doses PO, IV, or IM.

How supplied

Capsules: 75 or 150 mg.
Liquid: 75 mg/5 cc.
Ampoules: 300 or 600 mg vials, 150 mg/cc.

Adverse reactions

May cause pseudomembranous colitis, severe diarrhea, abdominal cramps, hypersensitivity, transient neutropenia, and jaundice.

Notes

Prescribe with caution in atopic individuals and patients with gastrointestinal disorders.
For IV infusions dilute to a concentration of no more than 6 mg/cc and infuse slowly.

▶ **CLOXACILLIN**

Usage

A drug of first choice for many penicillinase-producing staphylococcal infections.

▶ CLOXACILLIN (Cont.)

Dosage

Pediatric: 50–150 mg/kg/day in 4 doses PO.
Adult: 1–4 gm/day in 4 doses PO.

How supplied

Capsules: 250 mg and 500 mg.
Suspension: 125 mg/5 cc.

Adverse reactions

Same as with other penicillins.

Notes

Best absorbed on empty stomach, 1 hour before or after meals.
Other penicillinase-resistant penicillins include:
   Dicloxicillin (PO, dosage 1/2 that of cloxacillin)
   Methicillin (IV or IM)
   Nafcillin (IV or IM, dosage same as methicillin)
   Oxacillin (PO, dosage same as cloxacillin, IV, dosage same as methicillin).

▶ CO-TRIMOXAZOLE: TRIMETHOPRIM AND SULFAMETHOXAZOLE (BACTRIM, SEPTRA)

Usage

May be useful for *E. coli,* klebsiella, proteus, *Pneumocystis carinii, Salmonella typhi,* and shigella infections.
Often effective in chronic prostatitis and urinary tract infections.
Also approved for UTIs, pneumocystis, and otitis media in children.

Dosage

Pediatric: (Not recommended for newborns) 20 mg trimethoprim—100 mg
         sulfa/kg/day for severe infections.
Adult: 2 tablets bid.

How supplied

Tablets: Single strength—80 mg trimethoprim and 400 mg sulfamethoxazole
(double strength tablets available).
Liquid: 40 mg trimethoprim and 200 mg sulfamethoxazole/5 cc.

Adverse reactions

Frequent gastrointestinal disturbances and rashes. Occasional blood dyscrasias
and crystalluria.
Aggravates folate deficiency (may be reversed by treatment with folinic acid).

▶ CO-TRIMOXAZOLE
(TRIMETHOPRIM SULFAMETHOXAZOLE)
(Cont.)

Drug interactions

Tolbutamide: May cause hypoglycemia.
Methotrexate: Increases toxicity.
Anticoagulants: Increases anticoagulation.
Dilantin: Increases dilantin toxicity.
Thiazides: Increases chance of thrombocytopenia.

▶ DICLOXACILLIN (See Cloxacillin, equivalent drug)

Dosage

One-half that of cloxacillin.

How supplied

Capsules: 125, 250, and 500 mg.
Suspension: 62.5 mg/5 cc.

▶ ERYTHROMYCIN

Usage

A drug of choice for most *bordetella pertussis,* mycoplasma, Legionnaires' disease, and diphtheria infections. Also useful for pneumococcal, streptococcal, staphylococcal, and clostridial infections especially in penicillin-sensitive patients.

Dosage

Pediatric: 30–50 mg/kg/day in 4 doses PO.
         10 mg/kg/day in 3 doses IV or IM.
Adult: 1–4 gm/day in 4 doses IV, IM, or PO.

▶ **ERYTHROMYCIN (Cont.)**

How supplied

	Tablets	Capsules	Liquid	Drops	Vials
Stearate salt	125, 250, 500 mg	—	—	—	100 or 500 mg/vial
Ethyl succinate salt	200 or 400 (chewable)	—	200 or 400 mg/ 5 cc	—	2 cc and 10 cc vials (50 mg/cc for IM)
Estolate salt	125, 250 mg (chewable) 500 mg	125 or 250 mg	125 or 250 mg/ 5 cc	100 mg/ cc	—
Lactobionate	—	—	—	—	500 mg or 1 gm per vial (for IV)

Adverse reactions

Gastrointestinal disturbances common.
Stomatitis may occur.
IM injection is painful and IV infusion should be slow, over 20–60 minutes (thrombophlebitis is common).
Cholestatic jaundice may occur with estolate salt.

Notes

Staphylococcus aureus may develop resistance to erythromycin during treatment.

▶ **ETHAMBUTOL**

Usage

May be useful in multidrug regimen against tuberculosis.

Dosage

Pediatric: 15–20 mg/kg/day single dose PO (not recommended for use in children under 13).
Adult: Same, 15–25 mg/kg/day.

How supplied

Tablets: 100 and 400 mg.

Adverse reactions

Rarely, retrobulbar neuritis may occur (dose related if more than 25 mg/kg/day given). May cause hyperuricemia in predisposed patients.

▶ **GENTAMICIN**

Usage

A drug of choice for many enterobacter, proteus (indole pos.), pseudomonas, and serratia infections. May also be useful in *Streptococcus fecalis,* staphylococcus, klebsiella and *E. coli* infections. (See kanamycin and tobramycin.)

Dosage

Newborn: Under 1 week, 3–5 mg/kg/day in 2 doses IM or IV.
Pediatric: 5–7 mg/kg/day in 3 doses IM or IV.
Adult: 3–6 mg/kg/day in 3 doses IM or IV.

How supplied

Vials: 40 mg/cc (1.5-cc and 2-cc vials or 10 mg/cc in 2-cc vials). Also available as topical cream, ophthalmic solution, and ointment.

Adverse reactions

Occasional reports of vestibular and renal damage.
Hearing loss rare.

Drug interactions

Curare-type drugs: May increase neuromuscular blockade resulting in apnea.

Notes

Slow IV infusion is recommended. If available, monitor with blood levels.

▶ ISONIAZID (INH)

Usage

Useful in treatment of tuberculosis as part of multidrug regimen. Used alone as preventive therapy for contacts or those with positive skin tests who warrant therapy (see page 174).

Dosage

Pediatric: 10–15 mg/kg/day (up to 300 mg/day PO once a day).
Adult: 300 mg PO once a day.

How supplied

Tablets: 50, 100, 300 mg.
Capsules: 300 mg.
Liquid: 10 mg/cc (may cause diarrhea in this form).
Ampoules: 100 mg/cc (for IV or IM use).

Adverse reactions

Occasional peripheral neuropathy in diabetics, adolescents, and malnourished patients (preventable by giving B6 (pyrodoxine) 50–100 mg/day).
Hepatitis and gastrointestinal upset may occur in adults.

Drug interactions

Aluminum antacids: May inhibit gastrointestinal absorption of INH.
Rifampin: May increase INH hepatotoxicity.
PAS: May increase INH hepatotoxicity.
Diphenylhydantoin: May increase diphenylhydantoin toxicity, by reduced hepatic metabolism.

Notes

CSF levels: excellent.

▶ KANAMYCIN

Usage

Useful for enterobacter, *E. coli,* and serratia infections. May also be useful in brucella and proteus (indole pos.) infections.

Dosage

Newborn: Under 1 week or low birth weight (under 2000 gm), 20 mg/kg/day
in 2 doses IM.
1 week to 1 month, 30 mg/kg/day in 3 doses IM.
Pediatric: 15 mg/kg/day in 2 doses IM or IV.
Adult: 4–8 gm/day in 2 doses PO (for bowel sterilization);
10–15 mg/kg/day in 2 doses IM or IV (for infections).

▶ **KANAMYCIN (Cont.)**

How supplied

Capsules: 500 mg.
Ampoules: 0.5 gm in 2 cc, 0.75 gm in 2 cc, or 1 gm in 3 cc.

Adverse reactions

Ototoxicity and renal toxicity.

Drug interactions

Same as gentamicin.

Notes

IM is the preferred route of administration. When given IV, infusion should be very slow.

▶ **METHICILLIN**

Usage

For parenteral treatment of serious infections caused by penicillinase-producing *Staphylococcus aureus.*

Dosage

Newborn: Under 1 week, 50–100 mg/kg/day in 2 doses IV or IM.
Pediatric: 100–200 mg/kg/day in 4–6 doses IV or IM.
Adult: 4–12 gm/day in 4–6 doses IV or IM.

How supplied

Ampoules: 1, 4, or 6 mg vials.

Adverse reactions

Bacterial and/or fungal overgrowth may occur after prolonged use.
Reversible interstitial nephritis (may be dose-related).

Notes

Painful if given IM.

▶ **MINOCYCLINE**

Usage

Useful for many asymptomatic meningococcal carriers.

Dosage

Pediatric: 4 mg/kg first dose, then 4 mg/kg/day in 2 doses PO.
Adult: 200 mg first dose, then 200 mg/day in 2 doses PO.

▶ MINOCYCLINE (Cont.)

How supplied

Capsules: 50 and 100 mg.
Ampoules: 100 mg.
Syrup: 50 mg/5 cc.

Adverse reactions

Vertigo may occur.
See Tetracycline for other adverse reactions.

▶ NEOMYCIN

Usage

A drug of choice for suppression of intestinal bacteria in cases of hepatic coma,
diarrhea due to enteropathogenic *E. coli* in infants, and preoperative preparation
to bowel surgery.

Dosage

Pediatric: For enteropathic *E. coli* gastroenteritis—50–100 mg/kg/day in 4 doses
PO (neonate: same).
Adult: For prep prior to bowel surgery—40 mg/kg/day in 6 doses PO.
For hepatic coma, first day 100 mg/kg/day in 4 doses PO, thereafter
50 mg/kg/day.

How supplied

Tablets: 500 mg.
Liquid: 125 mg/5 cc.
Ampoules: 500 mg vial.
Ointments or powders.

Adverse reactions

Nephrotoxicity and ototoxicity (increased with concurrent use of ototoxic
diuretics).
Hypersensitivity, cross-sensitivity with other aminoglycosides (gentamicin,
kanamycin, streptomycin, tobramycin).

Drug interactions

Tubocurarine and succinyl choline: May increase neuromuscular blockade of
curariform drugs.
Ethacrynic acid: May enhance ototoxicity.

Notes

Poor gastrointestinal absorption.

▶ **NAFCILLIN**

Usage

Against penicillinase-producing staphylococci and pneumococci.

Dosage

Newborn: 30–40 mg/kg/day in 3 or 4 doses IV.
Pediatric: 25–50 mg/kg/day in 4 doses IV.
Adult: 100 mg/kg/day in 4 doses IV (maximum dose 6 gm/day).

Route of administration

IV, IM, and PO (see note below).

How supplied

Capsules and tablets: 250 mg and 500 mg.
Vials: 500 mg, 1 gm, and 2 gm.
Solution: 250 mg/5 cc with 2% alcohol in 80 cc bottle.

Adverse reactions

Similar to other penicillins.
Incidence of nephritis may be lower than with methicillin.

Drug interactions

Similar to other penicillins.

Notes

Not recommended for oral use because of erratic absorption.
Excreted mostly in bile, so adjustment in renal failure is not needed.

▶ **OXACILLIN***

Usage

Useful for many penicillinase-producing *Staphylococcus aureus* infections.
Best limited to parenteral use.

Dosage

Newborn: Under 1 week, 50 mg/kg/day in 2 doses IV or IM.
Pediatric: 50–150 mg/kg/day in 4 doses PO.
         100–300 mg/kg/day in 6 doses IV.
Adult: 1–6 gm/day in 4 doses PO.
         4–12 gm/day in 6 doses IV.

*See Methicillin or Nafcillin.

OXACILLIN (Cont.)

How supplied

Capsules: 250 and 500 mg.
Liquid: 250 mg/5 cc.
Vials: Variable concentrations.

▶ PARAAMINOSALICYLIC ACID (PAS)

Usage

May be useful in multidrug regimen against tuberculosis.

Dosage

Pediatric: 200–300 mg/kg/day in 3 doses PO.
Adult: Same—usually 8–12 gm/day in 3 doses PO.

How supplied

Tablets: 300 mg, 500 mg, 1 gm, 2 gm.

Adverse reaction

Liver damage and allergic reactions; nausea, vomiting, diarrhea, and abdominal pain may be reduced by administration with meals.

Drug interaction

INH: May increase INH blood levels or toxicity, by inhibiting breakdown.
Anticoagulants (bishydroxycoumarin): May increase anticoagulation, by inhibiting breakdown.
Rifampin: May interfere with PAS absorption.
Acid urine: May increase PAS crystalluria.

Notes

Sodium salt contains 108.9 mg Na+/gm.
Deteriorates with heat and sunlight.
If Na+, K+, or Ca++ salts are used rather than the acid form, doses must be adjusted at least 20% higher.

▶ PENICILLINS

Usage

Drugs of choice for most infections caused by betahemolytic streptococci, pneumococci, actinomyces, diphtheroides, meningococci, gonococci, clostridia, and anaerobic cocci, and syphilis, leptospirosis, and rheumatic fever prophylaxis.

▶ **PENICILLINS (Cont.)**

Adverse reactions

Maculopapular rash, urticaria, serum sickness-like reaction, anaphylaxis, convulsion, and platelet dysfunction.

▶ **PENICILLIN**
(AQUEOUS CRYSTALLINE PENICILLIN G)

Dosage*

Newborn: Under 1 week, 50,000–100,000 units/kg/day in 2 doses IV or IM;
           1 week to 1 month, 75,000–150,000 units/kg/day in 3 doses IV or IM.
Pediatric: 25,000–300,000 units kg/day in 4–6 doses IM or IV.
Adult: 3–24 million units/day in 4–12 doses IV or IM.

How supplied

As a powder, in vials of 1, 5, 10, and 20 million units.

Notes

Sodium Penicillin G has 1.8 mEq of Na+/million units. Potassium Penicillin G has 1.7 mEq of K+ and 0.3 mEq of Na+/million units.

▶ **PENICILLIN**
(BENZATHINE IM)

Dosage

Newborn: 50,000 units kg once IM.
Pediatric: 300,000 units in infants under 6.6 kg; otherwise, 600,000 units
           every month IM. (Adult dose after 6 years of age.)
Adult: 1.2 million units every month IM (for rheumatic fever prophylaxis).

How supplied

Vials containing 300,000 units/cc, or in cartridge needle units containing 1–4 cc, with 600,000 units/cc. Supplied alone as L-A Bicillin or in 50% combination with procaine penicillin as C-R Bicillin (600,000 units each or 900,000 units benzathine with 300,000 units procaine).

▶ **PENICILLIN**
(PHENOXYMETHYL or PENICILLIN V)

Dosage

Pediatric: 125–250 mg/day in 4 doses PO.
Adult: 250–500 mg/day in 4 doses PO.

*400,000 units = 250 mg.

▶ **PENICILLIN**
(PHENOXYMETHYL or PENICILLIN V)
(Cont.)

How supplied

Tablets: 125, 250, 500 mg.
Liquid: 125 or 250 mg/5 cc.

Notes

Best absorbed on empty stomach, 1 hour before or 2 hours after a meal.
More acid-stable than penicillin G.

▶ **PENICILLIN**
(PENICILLIN G, POTASSIUM)

Dosage*

Same as penicillin V.

How supplied

Tablets: 100, 200, 250, 400, or 800,000 units/tablet or 1 million units/tablet.
Suspension: 125, 250, 400, or 500,000 units/5 ml.

Notes

Very acid-labile and results in unpredictable blood levels.
Penicillin V is preferable.

▶ **PENICILLIN (PROCAINE G)**

Dosage

Newborn: 50,000 units/kg/day in a single dose IM.
Pediatric: 300,000–1.2 million units/day in a single dose IM.
Adult: 1.2 million units/day in 2 doses IM.

How supplied

Usually in 300,000 units/cc, 500,000 units/cc, or 600,000 units/cc vials.
Often in combination with benzathine penicillin as C-R Bicillin.

▶ **POLYMYXIN B**

Usage

May be useful for *Pseudomonas aeruginosa* and enteric infections when organism
is resistant to kanamycin and gentamicin.

*400,000 units = 250 mg.

▶ **POLYMYXIN B (Cont.)**

Dosage

Pediatric: 2–4 mg/kg/day in 4 doses IV or IM.
            10–20 mg/kg/day in 2 doses PO for enteric infections.
Adult: 2.5 mg/kg/day in 4 doses IV.

How supplied

Tablets: 25 and 50 mg.
Vial: 500,000 units = 63.7 mg.
Also available as ointments, creams, ophthalmic and otic solutions.

Adverse reactions

Nephrotoxic and ototoxic.
May cause electrolyte abnormalities in patients with severe gram-negative sepsis.
Neurotoxicity manifested by irritability, weakness, numbness of extremities, and blurring of vision.

Drug interactions

See Gentamicin.

Notes

For IV infusion, administer over 1 hour.

▶ **RIFAMPIN**

Usage

May be useful as part of multidrug therapy for tuberculosis, to treat patients with Hansen's disease, or to treat asymptomatic carriers of *Neisseria meningitidis.*

Dosage

Pediatric: 10–20 mg/kg/day in a single dose PO (not recommended for children
            under 5).
Adult: 600 mg/day in a single dose PO. Meningitis prophylaxis 300 mg bid x
        2 days.

How supplied

Capsules: 300 mg.

Adverse reactions

Gastrointestinal disturbances and dizziness may occur. Hepatotoxicity rare. May discolor body secretions (e.g., urine, sweat, etc.).

▶ **RIFAMPIN (Cont.)**

Drug interactions

By enhanced breakdown of:
Warfarin: May cause decreased anticoagulation.
Oral contraceptives: May cause decreased contraceptive effect.

Notes

CSF levels: Poor.
Food in stomach delays absorption.

▶ **SPECTINOMYCIN**

Usage

May be useful for gonorrhea if patients are allergic to penicillin, or if strains are resistant.

Dosage

Pediatric: Safety in children not established.
Adult: 2 gm, single dose (4 gm max.).

How supplied

Ampoules: 400 mg/cc in 5-cc or 10-cc vials.

Adverse reactions

Urticaria, nausea, chills, and fever.

Notes

May mask or delay symptoms of incubating syphilis.
Safety in pregnancy not established.

▶ **STREPTOMYCIN**

Usage

May be useful as part of multidrug therapy against tuberculosis, plague, tularemia.

Dosage

Pediatric: 20–40 mg/kg/day in a single daily dose IM.
Adult: 1–2 gm/day in a single daily dose IM.

How supplied

Ampoules: 0.5 gm/cc in 2-cc or 10-cc vials.

▶ STREPTOMYCIN (Cont.)

Adverse reactions

Ototoxicity (nausea, vomiting, vertigo), nephrotoxicity, visual disturbances, and neuromuscular blockade.

Drug interactions

See Gentamicin.

▶ SULFAMETHOXAZOLE

Usage

May be useful in *E. coli,* klebsiella-aerobacter, enterobacter UTIs, *Staphylococcus aureus* and *Proteus mirabilis* infections, as well as for prophylaxis of meningococcal meningitis when organism is known to be a sensitive, group A strain.

Dosage

Pediatric: 50 mg/kg/day in 2 doses PO (give daily dose as loading dose).
            (Not recommended for infants under 2 months of age.)
Adult: 2 gm/day in 2 doses PO (give loading dose of 2 gm).

How supplied

Tablets: 500 mg.
Liquid: 500 mg/5 cc.

Adverse reactions

Maculopapular and urticarial rashes.

Drug interactions

Tolbutamide: Hypoglycemia.
Methotrexate: Toxicity increased.
Anticoagulants: Anticoagulation increased.
Diphenylhydantoin: Toxicity increased.
Bilirubin: Kernicterus increased.
Phenylbutazone; aspirin; probenecid: May increase serum level and activity of sulfas.

Notes

Crystalluria is preventable with increased fluid intake.
Use with caution in patients with asthma, severe allergy, G6PD deficiency or intermittent porphyria.

▶ SULFISOXAZOLE

Usage

See Sulfamethoxazole.

Dosage

Note: Give loading dose of half total daily dosage.
Pediatric: 100–150 mg/kg/day in 4 doses PO.
           100 mg/kg/day in 4 doses IV (slowly over 1 hour).
Adult: 4 gm/day in 4 doses PO.

How supplied

Tablets: 500 mg.
Liquid: 500 mg/5 cc.
Ampoules: 400 mg/cc in 5-cc or 10-cc vials.

Notes

See Sulfamethoxazole.

▶ TETRACYCLINES

Usage

A drug of choice for many brucella, plague, borellea, cholera, mycoplasma, chlamydia, rickettsia, and psittacosis infections.
May also be useful in gonococcal, syphillitic, pasteurella, and anaerobic infections. Rarely indicated in children (see adverse reactions below).

Dosage

Pediatric: 20–40 mg/kg/day in 4 doses PO, IV, or IM.
Adult: 1–2 gm/day in 4 doses PO, IV, or IM.

How supplied

Ampoules: 250 mg/vial.
Liquid: 125 mg/5 cc and 250 mg/5 cc.
Capsules: 250, 500 mg.
Drops: 100 mg/cc.
Also available in topical ointment and opthalmic preparations.

Adverse reactions

Gastrointestinal disturbances, photosensitivity, liver damage, prerenal azotemia, blood dyscrasias, overgrowth of monilia, and resistant organisms.
Discolors teeth in children under age 8.

▶ **TETRACYCLINES (Cont.)**

Drug interactions

Barbiturates and anticonvulsants: Cause increased doxycycline metabolism. (See Notes below.)

Notes

Give at least 1 hour before and 2 hours after meals.
Do not give with milk, antacids, or oral iron.
Doxycycline is a long-acting tetracycline (dose 100–200 mg PO or IV in a single daily dose).

▶ **TOBRAMYCIN**

Usage

Useful for most pseudomonas, proteus, *E. coli,* klebsiella, citrobacter, and staphylococcal infections.

Dosage

Pediatric: 3–5 mg/kg/day in 3 doses IM or IV (neonates under 1 week of age: 4 mg/kg/day in 2 doses IM or IV).
Adult: 3–5 mg/kg/day in 3 doses IM or IV.

How supplied

Ampoules: 10 mg/cc and 40 mg/cc (2-cc vials).
Disposable syringes: 60 mg/1.5 cc and 80 mg/2cc.

Adverse reactions

Ototoxicity, nephrotoxicity.

Drug interactions

See Gentamicin.

Notes

Cross-allergenicity with other aminoglycosides (e.g., gentamicin, amikacin).

▶ **VANCOMYCIN**

Usage

May be useful for methicillin-resistant staphylococcal infections and enterococcal endocarditis in penicillin-allergic patients. Effective against gonococci, coryne-bacteria, and clostridia.

▶ VANCOMYCIN (Cont.)

Dosage

Pediatric: 40 mg/kg/day in 2–4 doses IV slowly (give each dose over 30 minutes). Newborn and premature infants, 10 mg/kg/day in 2 doses IV.
Adult: 2 gm/day in 4 doses IV slowly.

How supplied

Ampoules: 500 mg/10 cc.
Powder for oral use: 10 gm.

Adverse reactions

Frequent chills, fever, nausea, and skin reactions.
Ototoxicity, nephrotoxicity, and tissue necrosis (if given IM) may occur.

ANTIPARASITICS

▶ CHLOROQUINE PHOSPHATE (ARALEN)

Usage

Malaria and amebiasis (hepatic abscess).

Dosage

Pediatric: 5 mg base/kg/day PO max.
Adult: 1 gm (2 tablets)/day PO max.
Note: Check each disease for indicated dose and schedule.

How supplied

Tablets: 500 mg chloroquine phosphate (= 300 mg base).
Note: Chloroquine HCl is a different preparation, with similar usage.

Adverse reactions

Pruritus, vomiting, headaches.

Notes

Prolonged use may cause keratopathy, retinopathy, or visual disturbances. Ocular toxicity is dose-related and retinopathy is irreversible unless treatment is stopped upon early detection.

▶ **CROTAMITON (EURAX 10%)**

Usage

Scabies.

Dosage

Apply a thin layer uniformly and massage gently into all skin surfaces avoiding the face, eyes, mucous membranes, or any acutely inflamed skin or weeping surfaces. Apply again after 24 hours and wash off 48 hours after last application to remove drug. Treatment may be repeated in 7–10 days.

How applied

Cream: 60-gm tube.
Lotion: 6 oz and 16 oz.

Adverse reactions

Slight local irritation, particularly of face, eyes, or mucous membranes.

Notes

Pruritus may continue after treatment with drug. This is not an indication of treatment failure, but of acquired sensitivity to mites and their products.

▶ **DIIODOHYDROXYQUINOLINE**

Usage

Effective against both trophozoite and cyst forms of *Entamoeba histolytica.* Principally used against intestinal amebiasis or in combination with another amebicide in treatment of acute amoebic dysentery. Also effective locally against *Trichomonas vaginalis.*

Dosage

Pediatric: 90–120 mg/kg/day for 20 days (max. 6 gm/day).
Adult: 650 mg tid x 20 days (for asymptomatic cyst passers).

How supplied

650-mg tablets.

Adverse reactions

Abdominal distress, diarrhea, or constipation.

Drug interactions

May increase PBI and I^{131} uptake (thyroid function tests).

▶ **DIIODOHYDROXYQUINOLINE (Cont.)**

Notes

Use with caution in patients with iodine intolerance, severe thyroid disease, or hepatic or renal damage.

Possibility of iodism should be kept in mind.

▶ **GAMMA BENZENE HEXACHLORIDE (LINDANE or KWELL)**

Usage

Head, body, and pubic lice, and scabies.

Dosage

Apply topically on affected areas, wash off in 12–24 hours, reapply in 7 days if necessary.

How supplied

Cream: 2-oz tubes, 1-lb jars.
Lotion: 2 or 16 fluid oz, 1 gallon.
Shampoo: In bottles 2 oz, 16 fl oz, or 1 gallon.

Adverse reactions

Eczematous eruptions in sensitized patients.

Drug interactions

None reported.

Notes

Repeated or excess use may cause neurotoxicity.

▶ **MEBENDAZOLE (VERMOX)**

Usage

Whipworm, pinworm, ascaris, and hookworm infestations.

Dosage

Pediatric: For pinworms—100 mg PO single dose.
　　　　　For whipworms, ascaris, and hookworms—300 mg/day PO in 3 doses
　　　　　x 3 days. (Not recommended for children under 2 yrs.)
Adult: Same as pediatric.

▶ MEBENDAZOLE (VERMOX)
(Cont.)

How supplied

Chewable tablets: 100 mg.

Adverse reactions

Abdominal pain and diarrhea.

Drug interactions

None known.

Notes

Contraindicated in pregnant women.
Little experience in children under 2 years.

▶ METRONIDAZOLE (FLAGYL)

Usage

Giardiasis, trichomoniasis, amebiasis, *H. vaginalis* vaginitis.

Dosage

Pediatric: 15 mg/kg/day PO in 3 doses (750 mg/day max.)
Adult: For giardiasis or trichomoniasis—750 mg/day PO in 3 doses x 10 days
(1 tablet tid).
For amebiasis, intestinal—2250 mg (9 tablets)/day PO in 3 doses x 5–10
days.

How supplied

Tablets: 250 mg.

Adverse reactions

Nausea, headache, dry mouth, metallic taste.

Drug interactions

Antabuse-like reactions if taken with alcohol.

Notes

Contraindicated during first trimester of pregnancy.
If used during lactation, temporarily select alternate infant feeding method.

▶ NICLOSAMIDE

Usage

Effective against tapeworms.

Dosage

Pediatric: 11–34 kg–1 gm/kg/day x 5 days.
  Over 34 kg–1.5 gm/mg/day x 5 days.
Adult: 2 gm in 2 doses, 1 hour apart.

How supplied

500-mg chewable tablets.

Adverse reactions

Minimal.

Drug interactions

Minimal.

Notes

Tablet must be chewed thoroughly before swallowing and washed down with water. Patient should abstain from solid food on the evening before treatment. The next morning, a dose of 1 gm is given on an empty stomach, followed 1 hour later by another dose of 1 gm. A meal may be taken 2 hours thereafter. A brisk purgative is recommended 2 hours after the last dose to expel the worms and to minimize the possibility of the migration of the ova into the stomach with the consequent risk of cysticercosis.

Clinical cure cannot be assessed for 3 months since the drug causes worm digestion and the scolex is rarely identified posttreatment.

▶ NIRIDAZOLE (AMBILHAR)

Usage

Useful in schistosomiasis (especially due to *S. haematobium*) and amebiasis.

Dosage

Pediatric: May receive up to 35 mg/kg/day in 2 doses PO x 5–7 days.
Adult: 25 mg/kg/day (maximum dose of 1.5 gm/day) in 2 doses PO x 5–7 days.

How supplied

Tablets: 100 mg and 500 mg.

▶ **NIRIDAZOLE (AMBILHAR)**
(Cont.)

Adverse reactions

Anorexia, nausea and vomiting, diarrhea, dizziness, headache, and abdominal pain. Hemolysis may occur in those with G6PD deficiency. Children tolerate side-effects better.

Drug interactions

Minimal.

Notes

Use with caution in patients with hepatic impairment.
May be contraindicated in patients with epilepsy, severe heart disease, or a history of mental disturbance.
Discolors urine dark brown.

▶ **PIPERAZINE CITRATE (ANTEPAR)**

Usage

Ascaris and pinworm infestations.

Dosage

Pediatric: 75 mg/kg/day PO (single dose) x 2 days (max. 3.5 gm/day).
Adult: 3.5 gm/day PO (single dose) x 2 days.

How supplied

Tablets: 500 mg.
Syrup: 500 mg/5 cc.

Adverse reactions

Dizziness, neurotoxicity, hypersensitivity reactions, and gastrointestinal disturbance occasionally occur.

Notes

Avoid repeated treatment in excess of recommended dose.

▶ **PRIMAQUINE**

Usage

Specific activity against exo-erythrocytic or tissue forms of malaria (*Plasmodium vivax, P. ovale*). Used for chemoprophylaxis. (*Note:* Not satisfactory alone for acute malaria, but valuable in relapsing malaria).

▶ PRIMAQUINE (Cont.)

Dosage

Pediatric: 0.3 mg (base)/kg/day in single dose x 14 days.
Adult: 15 mg (base)/day in single dose x 14 days or 45 mg/week x 8 weeks.

How supplied

26.3-mg tablets (= 15 mg base).

Adverse reactions

Mild to moderate abdominal cramps and epigastric distress may be alleviated by antacids or by taking the drug at mealtime. Hemolytic anemia may occur in patients with G6PD deficiency.

▶ PYRANTEL PAMOATE (ANTEMINTH)

Usage

Hookworm, pinworm, and ascaris infestations.

Dosage

Pediatric: 11 mg/kg (max. 1 gm) single dose PO.
Adult: Same as pediatric.
Note: Same as 5 mg/lb, or 1 ml suspension/10 lb.

How supplied

Oral suspension: 50 mg/ml in 60-ml bottles.

Adverse reactions

Nausea, vomiting, anorexia, headache, dizziness, rash, fever, are frequent.

Drug interactions

None reported.

Notes

Little experience in pregnant women or children under age 2.

▶ PYRVINIUM PAMOATE (POVAN)

Usage

Pinworm infestations.

▶ **PYRVINIUM PAMOATE (POVAN)**
(Cont.)

Dosage

Pediatric: 5 mg/kg/day (max. 250 mg) single dose PO, repeat in 2 weeks if necessary.
Adult: Same as pediatric.

How supplied

Tablets: 50 mg.
Suspension: 10 mg/ml in 2-oz bottles.

Adverse reactions

Turns stool red, vomiting, diarrhea.

Notes

Unknown risks for pregnant women.
Advise patient of staining properties.
Tartrazine, the dye in the tablet coating, may cause allergic reactions.

▶ **QUINACRINE HYDROCHLORIDE**
(ATABRINE)

Usage

Giardiasis and cestodiasis (tapeworm infestations).

Dosage

For treatment of giardiasis:

Pediatric: 6 mg/kg/day PO (max. 300 mg/day) in 3 doses x 6 days.
Adult: 300 mg/day in 3 doses x 6 days.

Adverse reactions

Gastrointestinal complaints, toxic psychosis, blood dyscrasias, urticaria, dermatitis, transient headache and dizziness, and ocular effects.

Drug interactions

Primaquine: May increase primaquine toxicity.
Hepatotoxic drugs (e.g., alcohol, INH): May increase hepatotoxicity.

Notes

Take after meals with full glass of water, tea, or juice.
May cause temporary yellow discoloration of skin.
Sodium bicarbonate (1 gm) administered simultaneously may decrease urinary excretion of drug.

▶ THIABENDAZOLE (MINTEZOL)

Usage

Strongyloides and possibly trichinosis.

Dosage

Pediatric: 50 mg/kg/day PO in 2 doses. For strongyloides treat for 2 days.
For trichinosis treat 5–7 days or until toxic effects occur.
Adult: Same as pediatric.

How supplied

Chewable tablet: 500 mg.
Suspension: 500 mg/5 ml in 4-oz bottles.

Adverse reactions

Nausea, vomiting, vertigo, leukopenia, crystalluria, dermatitis, hallucinations, and olfactory disturbances.

ANTIFUNGALS

▶ AMPHOTERICIN B

Usage

For life-threatening fungal infections only.

Dosage

Pediatric: A test dose of 1 mg diluted in 250 cc 5% dextrose infused over 2–4 hours is recommended, then followed by a starting dose of 0.20–0.25 mg/kg/day single dose IV slowly over 3–6 hours. If tolerated, increase daily by 0.3 mg/kg/day to maximum dose of 1 mg/kg/day or 1.5 mg/kg/day every other day.
Adult: Same as pediatric.

How supplied

Vials: 50 mg of powder. Dilute to 1 mg/10 cc D5W, as described by insert.

Adverse reactions

Fever, chills, anorexia, weight loss, and gastrointestinal disturbances are common. Renal damage, anemia (bone marrow suppression), hypokalemia and thrombophlebitis may occur.

Drug interaction

Curariform drugs: Increase neuromuscular blockade, by hypokalemia.
Digitalis: May increase digitalis toxicity, by hypokalemia.

▶ **AMPHOTERICIN B (Cont.)**

Notes

Monitor serum potassium creatinine and hematocrit weekly.
Drug is physically incompatible with diluents containing bacteriostatic agents or electrolytes (i.e., Na+, K+, Ca++, etc.).

▶ **CLOTRIMAZOLE (LOTRIMIN)**

Usage

Effective against fungi, yeasts, dermatophytes, some gram-positive bacteria, and *Trichomonas vaginalis.*

Dosage

Skin involvement: Apply topically on affected areas twice a day for at least 1 week.
Vaginitis: Insert 1 vaginal tablet each day for 7 days.

How supplied

Cream (1%): 15 gm and 30 gm.
Solution (1%): 10 cc and 30 cc.
Vaginal tablets: 100 mg.

Adverse reactions

Mild skin irritation (e.g., erythema, pruritus, burning).

Drug interactions

Minimal.

Notes

Contraindicated in patients with hypersensitivity. Safety for vaginal use in first trimester of pregnancy is unknown.

▶ **GRISEOFULVIN**

Usage

For severe dermatophytoses involving scalp or nails.

Dosage

Pediatric: 10 mg/kg/day in single dose PO.
Adult: 0.5-1 gm/day in single dose.

How supplied

Tablets: 125, 250, and 500 mg.
Liquid: 125 mg/5 cc.

▶ **GRISEOFULVIN (Cont.)**

Adverse reactions

Headaches are frequent, especially in combination with alcohol. Gastrointestinal disturbances, hypersensitivity rashes, and photosensitivity may occur.
May aggravate acute intermittent porphyria due to interference with porphyrin metabolism.

Drug interactions

Anticoagulants: Anticoagulation increased.

▶ **NYSTATIN**

Usage

For candidiasis.

Dosage

Pediatric: For oral infection—2–6 cc PO qid, half of dose in each side of mouth, and swallow.
Adult: For oral or intestinal infection—6 cc PO qid.
     For vaginal infection—1 vaginal tablet qid or bid x 2 weeks.

How supplied

Vaginal tablet: 100,000 units/tablet.
Tablets: 500,000 units.
Liquid: 100,000 units/cc in 60-cc bottles with calibrated dropper.
Also available as cream and ointment.

Adverse reactions

Nausea and vomiting may occur.

Notes

Not absorbed from gastrointestinal, skin, or mucosal surfaces.

▶ **MICONAZOLE**

Usage

Active against dermatophytes (trichophyton, epidermophyton, and microsporum species), yeasts (cryptococcal, pityrosporon and candida species), certain dimorphic fungi (histoplasma, blastomyces), aspergillosis.

Dosage

Vulvovaginal candidiasis: One 5-gm intravaginal application per day for 2 weeks.
Tinea pedis, cruris, and corporis: Apply cream sparingly and rub into the skin bid x 2 weeks.

▶ MICONAZOLE (Cont.)

How supplied

Cream (2%): 3 gm.
Vaginal cream (2%): 85 gm with 5-gm applicators.

Adverse reactions

Burning, itching, or irritation in some patients.

Drug reactions

Minimal.

Notes

Minimal absorption from intravaginal application: caution in first trimester of pregnancy.

▶ TOLNAFTATE (TINACTIN)

Usage

Active against dermatophytes (microsporum spp, trichophyton spp, some epidermophyton spp) but not against candida or aspergillus.

Dosage

Topical application of cream, powder, or solution on affected areas 2–3 times per day x 2–3 weeks.

How supplied

Cream (1%): 15–gm tube.
Powder (1%): 45-gm bottle.
Powder (1%): 120-gm aerosol.
Solution (1%): 10-cc squeeze bottle.

Adverse reactions

Slight local irritation especially when in contact with excoriated skin or eye. Sensitization may develop to other ingredients in the cream rather than to the drug itself.

Drug reactions

Minimal.

Notes

May be used in conjunction with wet compresses for exudative lesions or keratolytic agents for plantar lesions.

4

ANTIMICROBIAL THERAPY

BASIC PRINCIPLES OF ANTIMICROBIAL THERAPY

A. Evaluate the clinical situation carefully.
B. Collect all appropriate clinical specimens including cultures and smears.
C. Choose an antimicrobial agent only if clinically indicated.
- It is best to direct therapy against a suspected agent rather than against a clinical manifestation such as fever.
- Treatment can always be changed if laboratory results show that the presumptive diagnosis was incorrect.
- Always select the drug with the narrowest antimicrobial spectrum considered to be effective.
- Dosage and duration of treatment should be as short as possible and as low as possible within the therapeutic range.
- The route of administration of antimicrobials should be determined not only by the severity of the infection, but also patient convenience and compliance.
- Beware of potential adverse side-effects such as:
  a. development of resistant strains of organisms;
  b. change of normal flora causing patient to be more susceptible to super-infections by other resistant organisms;
  c. allergic, toxic, and idiosyncratic reactions;
  d. effects on the fetus in pregnant women;
  e. effects on nursing newborn infants;
  f. prolongation of carrier state.
D. Common reasons for failures in antimicrobial therapy:
- Patient factors:
  a. patient is not taking the drug;
  b. patient is taking the drug improperly;
  c. patient has poor host-resistance.
- Drug factors:
  a. drug has not reached site of infection;
  b. inadequate dose or duration of treatment;
  c. improper route of administration;
  d. drug not specific against etiologic agent.
- Factors of the organism:
  a. An organism other than the one isolated by the laboratory is responsible for the infection.
  b. Organism is resistant to the therapy.
  c. Organism is protected within an abscess.
  d. Superinfection may have occurred.

ANTIBIOTICS IN PREGNANT OR LACTATING WOMEN

Antibiotics should not be used in pregnant or lactating women unless they are absolutely required. Penicillin is the only antibiotic known to be safe. Tetracyclines, chloramphenicol, and sulfonamides are known to be harmful.

Antibiotic	Passes placenta	Harmful to fetus	Present in milk	Harmful to newborn
Penicillin G	Yes	No	Yes	No
Ampicillin	Yes	No	Yes	No?
Methicillin	Yes	No	Yes	No
Carbenicillin	Yes	No	Yes	No?
Tetracyclines	Yes	Yes	Yes	Yes
Chloramphenicol	Yes	?	Yes	Yes
Erythromycin	Yes	No	Yes	No?
Streptomycin	Yes	Yes (rare)	Yes	Yes
Sulfonamides	Yes	Yes[a]	Yes	Yes
Nitrofurantoin	Yes	No	Yes	No?
Cephalosporins	Yes	No	No?	No?
Gentamicin	Yes	?	?	?

? = Unknown

No? = Probably not, but data inconclusive

[a] = Third trimester

References: Sabath, in Charles (Ed.) *Obstetrical and Perinatal Infections*, Lea & Febiger, Philadelphia, 1973.

Eisenberg, Mickey and Ray, George C. *Manual of Antimicrobial Therapy and Communicable Diseases*, State of Washington, Department of Social and Health Services, 1976.

Vorher, Helmuth. "Drug Excretion in Breast Milk," *Postgrad. Med.* **56** (4): 97–104, Oct. 1974.

O'Brien. "Excretion of Drugs in Human Milk." *Nursing Digest*, 23–31, Aug. 1975.

ANTIMICROBIAL PROPHYLAXIS

▶ PREVENTION OF BACTERIAL ENDOCARDITIS

Prophylaxis is often used before dental or certain surgical procedures to prevent bacterial endocarditis in patients with valvular heart disease and other cardiac abnormalities.* There are no controlled studies in humans proving its effectiveness.

Doses in the table are for adults, and first dose should be given about *one hour* before the procedure.

DENTAL AND UPPER RESPIRATORY PROCEDURES

Parenteral
Aqueous penicillin G 1–2 million units IM or IV, *plus* procaine penicillin G 600,000 units IM, then penicillin V 500 mg q6h for 4 doses

Penicillin allergy
Vancomycin 1 gm IV infused over 30 minutes, then erythromycin 500 mg PO q6h for 4 doses

Oral
Penicillin V 2 gm PO, then 500 mg PO q6h for 4 doses

Penicillin allergy
Erythromycin 1 gm, then 500 mg PO q6h for 4 doses

GASTROINTESTINAL AND GENITOURINARY PROCEDURES

Parenteral
Aqueous penicillin G 2 million units IM or IV (or ampicillin 1–2 gm IM or IV), *plus* streptomycin 1 gm IM; both to be repeated once 12 hours later.

Penicillin allergy
Vancomycin 1 gm IV infused over 30 minutes, *plus* streptomycin 1 gm IM; both to be repeated once 12 hours later.

Oral
Ampicillin 3.5 gm plus probenecid 1 gm PO, then ampicillin 15 mg/kg q6h for 4 doses; in addition, streptomycin 1 gm IM to be repeated once 12 hours later.

Penicillin allergy
An oral regimen that does not include penicillin or ampicillin is not likely to be effective.

*Most forms of congenital heart disease (but not uncomplicated secundum atrial septal defect), idiopathic hypertrophic subaortic stenosis, and mitral valve prolapse syndrome.

▶ **PREVENTION OF MENINGOCOCCAL DISEASE IN CONTACTS**

Prophylaxis should be given as soon as possible, and is usually indicated only for household contacts.

Rifampin 10 mg/kg/q12h PO x 2 days (maximum daily dose, 600 mg); 5 mg/kg/q12 h x 2 days (infants under 1 year), *or*

Minocycline 2 mg/kg/day PO q12h x 5 days (high frequency of vestibular toxicity), *or*

Sulfonamides may be used (4–5 days) if strain known to be sensitive.

▶ **RHEUMATIC HEART DISEASE PATIENTS**

Bicillin 1.2 million units IM every month (0.6 million units up to age 10 years). This is the preferred method and has the least recurrence rate, *or*

Phenoxymethyl penicillin 250 mg PO bid, *or*

Sulfisoxazole 1 gm daily.

▶ **PROPHYLAXIS OF RECURRENT URINARY TRACT INFECTION**

Prior to prophylaxis, urine should be sterilized with an antibiotic shown to be appropriate by sensitivity testing. Prophylaxis is usually continued for 3–12 months with:

Half tablet trimethoprim-sulfamethoxazole daily, *or*

Nitrofurantoin 50 mg daily.

▶ **TUBERCULOSIS**

Recommended for recent skin test (PPD) converters under age 35, children with positive skin tests, household contacts of sputum-positive cases, and patients who are immunodeficient or on long-term steroid therapy and have been exposed to tuberculosis.

Use INH 300 mg/day PO (children: 10 mg/kg/day) in a single daily dose for 1 year.

Note: People over 35 years old have increased risk of hepatotoxicity.

▶ **CONTAMINATED WOUNDS**

Many traumatic wounds can be considered contaminated. It is justifiable to use "prophylactic" antibiotics especially in wounds to the hand or foot. Use:

A penicillinase-resistant penicillin such as oxacillin 500 mg PO qid x 5 days, or a cephalosporin such as cephalothin 250 mg PO qid x 5 days.

▶ **TRAVELERS' DIARRHEA**

Doxycycline may be of benefit in preventing *E. coli* gastroenteritis.

MANAGEMENT OF PENICILLIN ALLERGIES

▶ **IMMEDIATE REACTIONS
(WITHIN 20 MINUTES)**

Anaphylaxis with rhinitis, urticaria, wheezing, and laryngeal edema.

Treatment

Stop penicillin administration.
Tourniquet above injection site.
Epinephrine (1 : 1000); adult dose 0.3 cc subcut., IM, or IV.
Antihistamines IV (e.g., Benadryl 50 mg for adults).
Aminophylline, oxygen, normal saline, intubation, etc., as needed.

▶ **ACCELERATED REACTIONS (1–72 HOURS)**

Urticaria, usually self-limited

Treatment

Epinephrine and antihistamines, as above.
Penicillin may be continued only if absolutely necessary.

▶ **DELAYED REACTIONS
(MORE THAN 72 HOURS)**

Skin rashes, usually maculopapular and pruritic

Treatment

Symptomatic (e.g., antihistamines).
Penicillin may be continued only if necessary.

Serum sickness with fever, arthralgia, myalgia, rash, lymphadenopathy

Treatment

Aspirin, antihistamines, steroids (if severe).
Discontinue penicillin.

Fever alone

Treatment

Aspirin.
Discontinue penicillin.

Interstitial nephritis or hemolytic anemia

Treatment

Discontinue penicillin.

▶ SKIN TESTING FOR PENICILLIN ALLERGY*

Materials

1. Old penicillin G, 1000 units/cc (minor determinant mixture, MDM) diluted with normal saline and let stand 2 weeks.
2. Penicilloyl-polylysine (PPL).

Procedure

1. Scratch test with both mixtures.
2. Wait 15 minutes. Positive is *any reaction.*
3. If negative, use 0.02 cc intradermal test with both (and a saline control). Wait 15 minutes. Positive is wheal of 5 mm or larger than saline control.

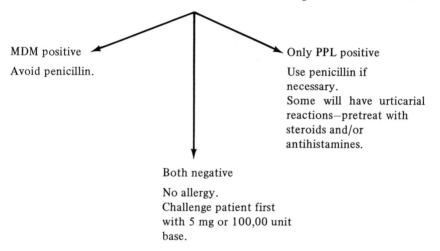

MDM positive

Avoid penicillin.

Only PPL positive

Use penicillin if necessary.
Some will have urticarial reactions—pretreat with steroids and/or antihistamines.

Both negative

No allergy.
Challenge patient first with 5 mg or 100,00 unit base.

*To be carried out only if adequate resuscitative drugs and equipment are available.

SUGGESTED ALTERATIONS OF MAINTENANCE DOSES DURING RENAL FAILURE*

Drug [a]	Normal dose (adults)	Normal dose interval	Degrees of renal failure — Mild [b]	Moderate [c]	Severe [d]	Significant Dialysis of drug [e]
Amphotericin	1 mg/kg/day	q24h	q24h	q24h	q24–36h	No (H) [e]
Celphalexin	0.25–1 gm	q6h	q6h	q6h (.25 gm)[f] q12h (.25 gm)	Yes (HP)	Yes (HP)
Cephalothin	1–2 gm	q4h	q4h	q6h	q8–12h (1 gm)	Yes (HP)
Cefazolin	0.5–1 gm	q8h	q12h	q12–16h (0.5 gm)	q24h (0.5 gm)	No (HP)
Ethambutol [g]	15 mg/kg/day	q24h	q24h (10 mg/kg)	q24h (5 mg/kg)	q24h (5 mg/kg)	Yes (HP)
Flucytosine	30–40 mg/kg	q6h	q6h	q12h	q24–36h	Yes (HP)
Gentamicin [h]	1–1.7 mg/kg	q8h	q8–12h	q12–24h	q48–72h	Yes (H) No (P)
Kanamycin [i]	7.5 mg/kg	q12h	q24h	q24–72h	q72–96h	Yes (HP)
Lincomycin	0.5 gm	q6h	q6h	q6h	q8–12h	No (HP)
Neomycin	1 gm (PO)	q6h	q6h	q12h	q18–24h	Yes (H) No (P)
Amoxicillin	0.25–1 gm	q8h	q8h	q12h	q16h (0.5 gm)	Yes (H)
Ampicillin	0.5–3 gm	q6h	q6h	q9h	q12–15h (1 gm)	Yes (H) No (P)
Carbenicillin	4–5 gm	q4h	q4h	q6–12h (2 gm)	q12–16h (2 gm)	Yes (H) No (P)

		Mild[b]	Moderate[c]	Severe[d]	
Methicillin	1–2 gm	q4h	q4h	q4h	q8-12h (1 gm)	No (HP)
Penicillin G	.25–4 million units	q4h	q4h (2 million units)	q4h (1.5 million units)	q6h (1 million units)	No (HP)
Pentamidine	4–5 mg/kg	q24h	q24h	q24–36h	q48h	Unknown
Quinine	650 mg	q8h	q8h	q8h	q12–16h	Yes (H) No (P)
Streptomycin	0.5 gm	q12h	q24h	q24–72h	q72–96h (0.5 gm)	Yes (HP)
Sulfa-Trimethoprim	1–2 tabs	q12h	q12h	q24h	Avoid	Yes (H)
Sulfisoxazole	1 gm	q6h	q6h	q8–12h	Avoid	Yes (HP)
Vancomycin	0.5–1 gm	q12h	q48–72h (0.5 gm)	q72–240h (0.5 gm)	q240h (0.5 gm)	No (HP)

*Adapted with permission from Eisenberg, Mickey and Ray, George C. *Manual of Antimicrobial Therapy and Communicable Diseases*. State of Washington, Department of Social and Health Services, 1976.

[a] The presence of an antibiotic on this list does *not* necessarily mean recommendation for use in renal failure.
[b] Mild renal failure: 50–80 ml/minute creatinine clearance.
[c] Moderate renal failure: 10–50 ml/minute creatinine clearance.
[d] Severe renal failure: less than 10 ml/minute creatinine clearance.
[e] (H) = hemodialysis; (P) = peritoneal dialysis.
[f] Maximum dose allowable.
[g] *Caution:* optic neuritis.
[h] Gentamicin formula: 1–1.5 mg/kg dose every (serum creatinine x 8) hours.
[i] Kanamycin formula: 7.5 mg/kg dose every (serum creatinine x 9) hours.

ANTIBIOTIC THERAPY IN PATIENTS WITH RENAL FAILURE*

Note: Avoid nephrotoxic drugs whenever possible.

TREATMENT OF UTIs: Use those agents which give adequate urine levels in spite of decreased renal function.

Adequate	*Inadequate*
Ampicillin	Chloramphenicol
Cephalothin	Nitrofurantoin
Cephalexin	Nalidixic acid
Gentamicin [a]	
Penicillin	
Tobramycin [a]	
Kanamycin [a]	

[a] Nephrotoxic

GUIDELINE FOR REDUCTION OF DOSAGE OF ANTIBIOTICS

Careful adjustment required	*Adjustment required only in severe renal failure*	*Little or no adjustment required*
Aminoglycosides[a]	Penicillin G	Cloxacillin
Carbenicillin	Ampicillin	Dicloxacillin
Cephalexin	Methicillin	Nafcillin
Cephaloridine	Oxacillin	Erythromycin
Colistin	Cephalothin	Doxycycline
Polymyxin B[b]	Cefazolin	Clindamycin
Tetracyclines	Lincomycin	Chloramphenicol
Nitrofurans	Trimethoprim-sulfa	Rifampin
Amphotericin B		Nalidixic acid
Ethambutol		Chloroquin
Flucytosine		Pryimethamine
		Isoniazid

[a] Nephrotoxicity potentiated by loop diuretics or cephalosporins.
[b] Except doxycycline.

*Adapted with permission from Eisenberg, Mickey and Ray, George C. *Manual of Antimicrobial Therapy and Communicable Diseases.* State of Washington, Department of Social and Health Services, 1976.

	AVERAGE WHOLESALE COSTS OF SOME ANTIMICROBIAL AGENTS	
Agent	*Average adult dose/day*	*Average wholesale cost/day to pharmacy*
Ampicillin	2 gm/day	$0.50
Amoxicillin	750 mg/day	1.00
Carbenicillin	2 gm/day	1.40
Cephalexin	1 gm/day	1.20
Cloxacillin	2 gm/day	1.80
Co-trimoxazole	4 tabs/day	0.85
Dicloxacillin	1 gm/day	1.00
Erythromycin stearate	1 gm/day	0.40
EES	1 gm/day	0.60
estolate	1 gm/day	0.85
Griseofulvin	1 gm/day	0.50
INH	300 mg/day	0.02
Kwell Lotion/Shampoo	2 oz	1.35
Mebendazole	100 mg/day	1.00
Metronidazole	750 mg/day	0.90
Nitrofurantoin capsules		
(macrocrystal)	100 mg/day	0.30
tablets	100 mg/day	0.05
Penicillin V	1 gm/day	0.16
Rifampin	600 mg/day	1.50
Sulfamethoxazole	2 gm/day	0.30
Sulfisoxazole	4 gm/day	0.35
Tetracyclines	1 mg/day	0.08

Note: The cost to the patient may be as much as 2–3 times that listed, and varies tremendously between pharmacies and geographic locales.

Reference: *American Druggist Blue Book*, October 1977, Updated Edition, The Hearst Corporation, New York, 1977.

5

THE LABORATORY

CONTENTS

GRAM STAIN IDENTIFICATION OF BACTERIA

▶ **TECHNIQUE**

1. Make thin smear of specimen. Air dry.
2. Heat fix (*not* too hot to touch). Let cool.
3. Flood with *crystal violet* 10 seconds. Rinse with tap water.
4. Flood with *Gram's iodine* 10 seconds. Rinse.
5. Decolorize with 95% ethanol, ethanol-acetone, or acetone alone until portion has no blue color. Rinse.
6. Flood with *Safranin* 10 seconds. Rinse. Blot or air-dry.

Note: Fluids should usually be spun before staining.
CSF incubation for 2 hours in a warm pocket may increase yield.
White cells and their nuclei should stain red.
If slide underdecolorized, repeat steps 5 and 6.
If slide overdecolorized, repeat steps 3 through 6.

	Bacilli (rods)	Pleomorphic organisms	Cocci	
Gram +	Clostridium Bacillus Lactobacillus	Corynebacterium Listeria	Streptococcus Staphylococcus *S. pneumoniae* Enterococcus spp.	Gram +

	Bacilli (rods)	Pleomorphic organisms	Cocci	
Gram −	Salmonella Shigella Pseudomonas *Escherichia coli* Proteus Aerobacter– Klebsiella Vibrio	Hemophilus Bacteroides Brucella Bordetella Mima-Herellea Pasteurella	Neisseria	Gram −

► BACTERIAL MORPHOLOGY— GRAM-NEGATIVE ORGANISMS

Gram-negative rods

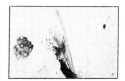 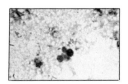 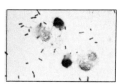

Klebsiella pneumoniae   *Pseudomonas aeruginosa*   *Escherichia coli*

Gram-negative pleomorphic

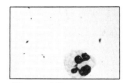 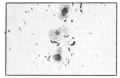 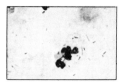

Hemophilus influenzae   *Hemophilus vaginalis*   *Bacteroides fragilis*

Gram-negative cocci

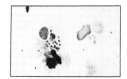 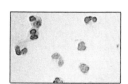

Neisseria gonorrhea   *Neisseria meningitidis*

Miscellaneous

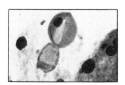 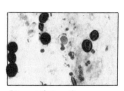

Stool artifact   Yeast (stool)

Normal flora

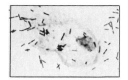 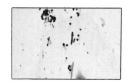

Vaginal discharge   Sputum

▶ **BACTERIAL MORPHOLOGY—
GRAM-POSITIVE ORGANISMS**

Gram-positive rods

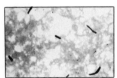

Clostridium tetani perfringens
or *botulinum*

Gram-positive cocci

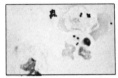

Staphyloccus aureus

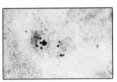

Streptococcus pyogenes

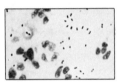

Streptococcus pneumoniae

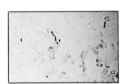

Enterococcus spp.

Gram-positive pleomorphic

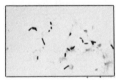

Listeria monocytogenes

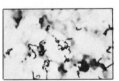

Corynebacterium diphtheriae
or diphtheroids

Miscellaneous

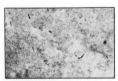

*Mycobacterium
tuberculosis*

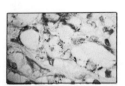

Mycobacterium leprae

CULTURE TECHNIQUES

Note: Always explain the procedure to the patient.

▶ THROAT CULTURE

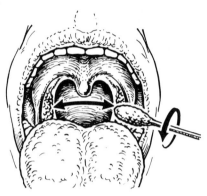

COMMENTS
• Rotate swab: touch both tonsils.

▶ CERVICAL CULTURE

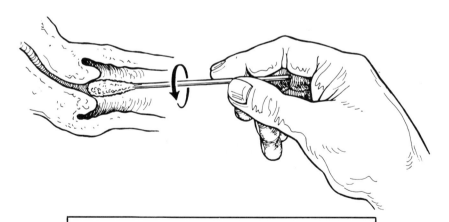

COMMENTS

• Rotate swab in cervical os.
• For gonorrhea also obtain an anal-canal culture and plate immediately.

▶ **BLOOD CULTURE**

Prep site

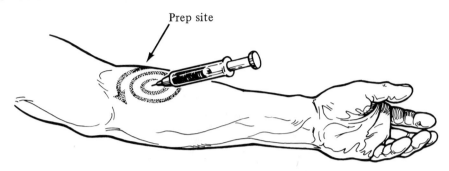

COMMENTS

- Prep site concentrically with iodine (if patient not hypersensitive) and alcohol.
- Use two separate sites for each of two samples.
- Collect 10 ml in adults and 1–2 ml in infants.
- Introduce air into bottle for aerobic specimen isolation.
- Blood to culture medium ratio of 1 : 10 to 1 : 20 is ideal.
- Mix contents to prevent clotting.
- Label aerobic and anaerobic bottles.

▶ **STOOL CULTURE**

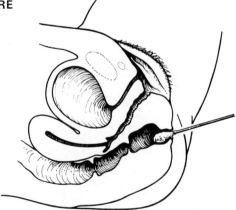

COMMENTS

- Best cultures are from stool samples, not rectal swabs.

▶ **SPINAL FLUID CULTURE**

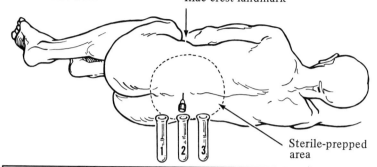

Iliac crest landmark

Sterile-prepped area

COMMENTS

- Position patient in knee-chest position. Sitting position may be helpful, especially for infants or children.
- Prep site carefully with iodine and then alcohol.
- Anesthetize area with 1% lidocaine. Avoid injecting into CSF space.
- Examine specimens for cells and bacteria. If none seen, incubate a specimen in a warm pocket for reexamination in 2 hours.
- Send samples to lab for smear, culture, and chemistries.
- Wipe excess iodine from skin site.

▶ **URETHRAL CULTURE**

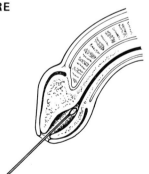

COMMENTS

- Use small urethral wire loop cotton swab.
- Prior massage of prostate may increase yield.
- If gonorrhea suspected, plant immediately.

▶ CONJUCTIVAL CULTURE

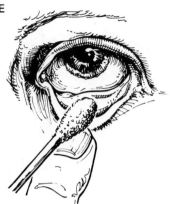

COMMENTS

- Obtain specimen from lower lid.
- Massage lacrimal duct if dacryocystitis suspected.

▶ URINE CULTURE

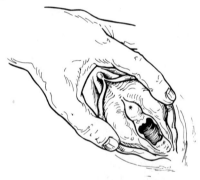

COMMENTS

For females:
- Prep vulvar area with soap and water.
- Collect midstream specimen while labia are held apart by patient.

- Refrigeration may stabilize bacterial counts for up to 24 hours.
- Urinary catheter tips are invariably contaminated.
- Suprapubic aspirate may be useful, especially in infants.

▶ STANDARD STREAK PLATE TECHNIQUE

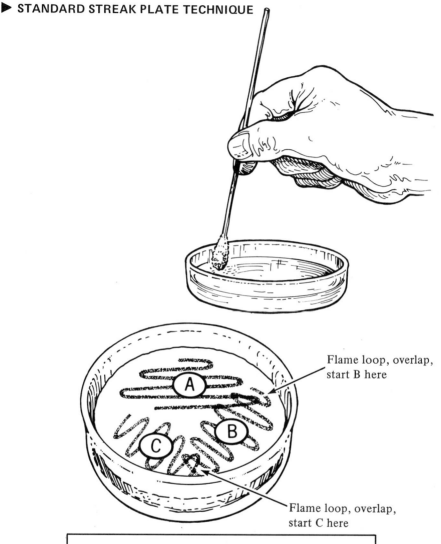

Flame loop, overlap, start B here

Flame loop, overlap, start C here

COMMENTS

- Streak swab or sterile loop with specimen in area A.
- Flame loop (without removing more inoculum) and allow to cool.
- Begin by streaking small part of A, then continue to area B.
- Flame loop again and allow to cool.
- Start on area B and progress to area C.
- Incubate petri plates upside down.

	RECOMMENDED TRANSPORT, ENRICHMENT, AND PLATING MEDIA FOR BACTERIAL ISOLATION			
Disease or Etiology	Transport	Enrichment	Plating	Remarks
Typhoid	Buffered glycerol saline Amies' Stuart's Cary-Blair	Selenite broth Tetrathionate broth	Bismuth sulfite agar SS agar MacConkey agar	Direct plating of fresh stools or rectal swabs preferred Hold and transport at room temperature or refrigerated
Salmonellosis	Tetrathionate brilliant green broth Buffered glycerol saline Cary-Blair Amies' Stuart's	Tetrathionate brilliant green broth Selenite broth Tetrathionate broth	Brilliant green agar Bismuth sulfite agar SS agar Xylose-lysine-deoxycholate (XLD) agar	May be transported in enrichment broth. Direct plating of specimens not recommended Hold and transport at room temperature or refrigerated
Shiga's bacillus dysentery	Cary-Blair Amies' Stuart's Buffered glycerol saline	None	Tergitol 7 agar XLD agar MacConkey agar	Direct plating of fresh stools or rectal swabs preferred Hold and transport at refrigerated temperature
Shigellosis (other than Shiga's bacillus)	Buffered glycerol saline Amies' Cary-Blair Stuart's	None	XLD agar SS agar Hektoen agar Deoxycholate citrate agar Tergitol 7 agar MacConkey agar	Direct plating of fresh stools or rectal swabs preferred Hold and transport at refrigerated temperature

Organism	Transport media		Special/selective media	Comments
E. coli	Amies' Stuart's Cary-Blair Buffered glycerol saline	Lactose broth Gram negative (GN) broth	MacConkey agar EMB agar Sheep blood (5%) TSA	Direct plating of stools preferred. Hold and transport at room temperature or refrigerated
Cholera	Cary-Blair Sea salt broth Monsur (bile peptone)	Alkaline peptone water Monsur's alkaline bile peptone water	Thiosulfate citrate bile salts (TCBS) agar Gelatin agar	Transport media are held and shipped at room temperature or refrigerated
Vibrio para-haemolyticus **gastroenteritis**	Cary-Blair	Peptone broth with 4% NaCl	TCBS agar	Halophilic organism—requires 3% NaCl for growth. Transport media held and shipped at room temperature or refrigerated
Corynebacterium diphtheriae	Pai Loeffler's Silica gel	Pai Loeffler's	Cystine tellurite blood agar Tinsdale agar	Preincubate Pai and Loeffler's 1 day at 37C before transporting
Gram negative (pseudomonas, klebsiella, enterobacter, proteus, etc.)	BHIB [a] TSB [b] Amies' Cary-Blair Stuart's	Brain heart infusion with 0.05% beef extract (BHIBE) BHIBE with neutralizers GN broth	MacConkey agar EMB agar Sheep blood (5%) TSA [c] Special selective media	Transport unincubated

Media listed in order of preference.
[a] BHIB = Brain heart infusion broth.
[b] TSB = Trypticase soy broth.
[c] TSA = Trypticase soy agar.

(Continued on next page)

RECOMMENDED TRANSPORT, ENRICHMENT, AND PLATING MEDIA FOR BACTERIAL ISOLATION (Cont.)

Disease or etiology	Transport	Enrichment	Plating	Remarks
Clostridium perfringens	Amies' Stuart's Cary-Blair	Cooked meat medium Thioglycolate broth	Egg yolk agar Blood agar SPS agar	Should use SPS agar for direct plate count on food. Transport media are held and shipped refrigerated
Staphylococcus	Trypticase soy agar plates (TSA) Amies' Stuart's Cary-Blair	TSB with 7% salt	TSA Sheep blood (5%) TSA Mannitol salt agar Staph 110 agar	Either Staph 110 agar or mannitol salts agar should be used for plating foods Transport media are held and shipped at room temperature
Meningococcus	Transgrow Modified Thayer-Martin agar	None	Modified Thayer-Martin agar	Incubated in candle jar or with 5% CO_2 Hold and transport at room temperature
Streptococcus	Silica gel Dry swab	BHI 0–2 hours incubation if swab is fresh but 4–5 hours incubation if in transport more than 8 hours	Sheep blood (5%) TSA	Fluorescent antibody methods are very good. Enrichment culture must be centrifuged and resuspended in 0.5 ml saline for FA smear preparation. Hold and transport at room temperature.

Hemophilus	Peptic digest broth BHI with growth factors	Peptic digest broth BHI with growth factors	Peptic digest agar Chocolate agar Rabbit blood (5%) TSA	Preincubate media before transport. Ship at room temperature.
Leptospira	Ellinghausen's Fletcher's	Ellinghausen's Fletcher's	None	Incubate at 28C 200 μg 5-fluorouracil/ml added to suppress contaminants. May be held and shipped at room temperature
Yersinia enterocolitica	Buffered saline Cary-Blair	Buffered saline	MacConkey agar SS agar	Incubate plates at 25C. Enrich in buffered saline at 4C for 4 weeks Hold and transport at 4C
B. pertussis	Casamine acid (2 hours) Bordet-Gengou	None	Bordet-Gengou	Sensitive to dehydration (incubate in moist atmosphere and seal plates for shipment)

Media listed in order of preference.
[a] BHIB = Brain heart infusion broth.
[b] TSB = Trypticase soy broth.
[c] TSA = Trypticase soy agar.

BLOOD FILM
PREPARATION

▶ **GENERAL COMMENTS**

Blood and other tissue smears may be useful in diagnosing malaria, trypanosomiasis, filiariasis, and other diseases caused by blood parasites.
Fresh blood is preferable to citrated, oxalated, or clotted blood.

Blood film preparation

Prepare finger or ear with gauze (not cotton).
Clean with 70% alcohol, allow to dry, and prick.
Allow films to dry in horizontal position.

Thin film

Deposit small drop on end of slide.
Spread with edge of cover slip or another slide.

Thick film (best for screening for parasites)

Touch the undersurface of the slide to a large drop of blood on the finger.
Do not touch the skin.
Rotate the slide to form a film about the size of a dime.

Whole blood

If concentration methods are to be used, collect blood aseptically by venipuncture, and add sodium citrate or heparin to prevent clotting.
Do not use preservatives.

Timing collection of specimen

In malaria this is important. Parasites are most numerous midway between chills, but their morphology at that time is somewhat less characteristic than it is later.
One specimen taken at this time and a second 5–6 hours later is ideal.

Storage of specimens

Prompt examination of specimens is best.
Unstained slides may be refrigerated for a week, but lose their affinity for stain after 3–4 days.
If staining is to be delayed, fix tissue and *thin films* with methyl alcohol and dehomoglobinize *thick films* in buffered water before storage. (Subsequent staining requires special technique.)
Refrigerate whole blood if not to be examined immediately (microfilariae remain alive in blood for a week or more under refrigeration).
Preserve stained blood films or other smears by covering with a coverslip or a coating of clear Diaphane or other neutral mounting medium.

WRIGHT STAIN FOR IDENTIFICATION
OF WHITE BLOOD CELLS AND BLOOD PARASITES

▶ **TECHNIQUE**

1. Air dry blood smear.
2. Flood slide with Wright stain.
3. Let stand 3 minutes.
4. Add buffer or water and mix by blowing until metallic green color appears.
5. Let stand horizontal about 7 minutes (depends on strength of stain).
6. Wash well with water *while horizontal* (to prevent precipitation of stain).
7. Air dry.
8. If stain is too light, reapply stain *and* buffer for several minutes.

NORMAL FLORA

▶ **GASTROINTESTINAL TRACT**

Large intestine (10^{11} bacteria/gm of contents)

Bacteroides
Diphtheroids
Coliforms (*Escherichia
    coli, Enterobacter
    aerogenes,* klebsiella)
Enterococci
Staphylococci
    (coagulase-positive and
    coagulase-negative)
Lactobacillus acidophilus
    and *brevis*

Spirochetes
Yeasts (candida, geotrichum,
    cryptococcus, penicillium,
    aspergillus)
Proteus
Pseudomonas
Bacillus subtilis
Actinomyces
Borrelia
Fusobacterium
Clostridium spp.

Breast-fed infants

L. bifidus (bifidobacterium)
Enterococci and coliforms (few)
Staphylococci (few)

Bottle-fed infants

L. acidophilus
Coliforms
Enterococci

Bacillus spp.
Clostridium spp.

Meconium

Usually sterile

▶ **NORMAL VOIDED URINE**

Usually sterile or less than 1000 colonies/ml. The following organisms are most often found in normal urine and are probably "contaminants" from the urethra and adjacent areas.

Staphylococcus epidermidis
Diphtheroids
Coliforms
Enterococci
Proteus spp.

Lactobacilli
Streptococci
   (alpha and beta-hemolytic)
Yeasts
Bacillus spp.

▶ **VAGINA**

Adult

L. acidophilus
S. epidermidis
Streptococci (alpha-hemolytic
   and nonhemolytic)
E. coli

Diphtheroids
Yeasts
Anaerobic streptococci
Listeria spp.
Clostridium spp.

▶ **SKIN**

S. epidermidis
S. aureus
Sarcina
Coliforms
Proteus
Diphtheroids
B. subtilis

Mycobacteria (external auditory canal,
   genital and axillary regions)
Candida albicans
Cryptococci
Streptococci (viridans group)
Enterococci
Mima

▶ **ORAL CAVITY**

At birth

Flora corresponds to organisms in mother's vagina (usually a mixture of micrococci, streptococci, coliforms, and L. acidophilus).

▶ ORAL CAVITY (Cont.)

After newborn period

Alpha-hemolytic streptococci
  (viridans group)
Neisseria catarrhalis
S. epidermidis
Haemophilus hemolyticus
Streptococcus pneumoniae
Nonhemolytic streptococci
Diphtheroids
Coliforms
Betahemolytic streptococci
  other than group A
Micrococci

Veillonella
Borrelia (*buccalis,*
  B. vincentii)
Fusobacterium
Actinomyces israelii
Yeasts (*C. albicans, geotrichum*)
Leptotrichia buccalis
Eikenella corrodens
Anaerobic micrococci
Anaerobic streptococci
Vibrios (anaerobic)
Spirochetes (*Treponema microdentium*)

▶ RESPIRATORY TRACT

Nasal passages

Diphtheroids
S. epidermidis
S. aureus
  (20–80% of population)
S. pneumoniae
  (5–15% of population)

Haemophilus influenzae
  (5–10% of population)
Neisseria spp.
  (0–15% of population)
N. meningitidis
  (0–4% of population)
Streptococci

Nasopharynx

(Sterile at birth)
Streptococci (viridans
  group)
Nonhemolytic streptococci
Neisseria spp.
  (90–100% of population)
Staphylococci (few)
H. influenzae
  (40–80% of population)
S. pneumoniae
  (20–40% of population)

Betahemolytic streptococci
  (5–15% of population)
N. meningitidis
  (5–20% of population)
H. parainfluenzae
Pseudomonas aeruginosa
E. coli
Proteus spp.
Paracolons
Diphtheroids
Bacteroides

Trachea, bronchi, lungs, and sinuses

Normally sterile

SPECIMENS FOR ISOLATION OF MYCOBACTERIA OR PATHOGENIC FUNGI (TUBERCULOSIS, HISTOPLASMOSIS)

Sputum

Collect 2–10 cc of material brought up from the lungs after productive cough or aerosolized saline inhalation. (Do not collect sputum immediately after a mouthwash.) A series (3) of single early-morning specimens, each shipped promptly to the laboratory after collection, is generally preferred to a pooled 24- or 48-hour specimen.

Gastric lavage

Gastric specimens should be collected early in the morning on a fasting stomach. Only sterile water should be used for collection. Examine within 4 hours. If specimens must be mailed, neutralize at the time of collection with buffer tablets or the addition of 10% sodium carbonate (50 mg).

Urine

First morning, clean-void midstream specimens are preferred over 24-hour collection because they are less likely to be contaminated.

Surgical or biopsy specimen

Collect and transport using aseptic technique. Protect viability of tissue by using sterile saline for transport.

SPECIMENS FOR ISOLATION OF VIRUSES

▶ GENERAL PRINCIPLES

Collect specimens as soon as possible after onset of illness.
Use sterile screw-capped or rubber-stoppered glass tube whenever possible (seal with adhesive tape).
Refrigerate (4C) or preferably freeze (−50C to −70C) as soon as possible.
Do *not* freeze specimens for herpes, CMV, or rabies.
Deliver or send to laboratory as soon as possible, in cold or frozen state.

Throat or rectal swabs

Swab throat and nasopharynx or rectum with swab moistened with buffered bacterial broth or balanced salt solution containing albumin. Freeze.

Urine

Collect 10–20 ml of clean void sample. *Note:* Do not freeze specimen for CMV.

Stool

Collect 1–2 teaspoonsful in 1-oz glass bottle. Use of cardboard containers for shipment tends to dry out specimens. Stool specimen may be mailed without refrigeration in standard virus isolation specimen mailing kit.

Spinal fluid

Collect 3–5 ml. Freeze, in slanted position.

Brain (for rabies)

Place head of animal into a suitable watertight metal container. Pack container in cracked ice in a larger watertight container (such as a metal cold-drink or picnic chest). Do *not* freeze. The following information is desirable when animal specimens are received for examination: the species; whether the animal died or was killed, and if killed, the means used; whether the animal was confined and observed before death; any symptoms of rabies; and a history of rabies vaccination.

Tissue specimen

Virtually any tissue can be used. Samples about 1/2–1 inch cubed are best. In cases of CNS involvement, submit samples of medulla, midbrain, temporal lobe cortex, and spinal cord. A 2–3 inch segment of descending colon, tied off with contents, should be included for the recovery of enteroviruses. For influenza or other respiratory disease, include sample of lung tissue and bronchus or trachea. Heart muscle, liver, and kidney are less common sources of virus but may be included if involvement is suspected.

APPROPRIATE SPECIMENS FOR VIRUS ISOLATION

Disease category agents generally sought	Throat	Stool	CSF	Urine	Vesicle[a] fluid	Other
Meningitis-encephalitis						
Mumps	++++	− −	++	+	− −	− −
Enteroviruses	+++	++++	+	− −	− −	− −
Herpes simplex	$\pm$	− −	$\pm$	− −	+	Brain biopsy +++
Arboviruses	− −	− −	+	− −	− −	Brain ++ Blood +
Respiratory diseases						
Myxoviruses						
Paramyxoviruses	++++	− −	− −	− −	− −	
Rhinoviruses						
Adenoviruses	++++	++++	− −	− −	− −	
Enteroviruses						
Exanthems						
Rubella[a]	++++	− −	− −	+	− −	
Rubeola [a]						
Variola [b]	++	− −	$\pm$	+	++++	
Vaccinia [b]	− −	− −	− −	− −	++++	
Varicella [b]	− −	− −	− −	− −	++++	
Herpes simplex [b]	++	− −	− −	− −	++++	
Enteroviruses [a]	+++	++++	− −	− −	+	
Myocarditis-pericarditis						
Enteroviruses [a]	++	+++	− −	− −	− −	Pericardial fluid ++
Myxoviruses[a]	+++	− −	− −	− −	− −	
Paramyxoviruses[a]	+++	− −	− −	− −	− −	
Other						
Cytomegalovirus	++	− −	− −	++++	− −	Leukocytes +

[a] Do not prep skin with alcohol or iodine.
[b] It is often difficult to isolate and/or associate these agents with the disease in question. Serologic tests are important to insure a diagnosis.

Adapted with permission from Eisenberg, Mickey and Ray, George C. *Manual of Antimicrobial Therapy and Communicable Diseases.* State of Washington, Department of Social and Health Services, 1976.

SPECIMENS FOR IDENTIFICATION
OF INTESTINAL PARASITES

▶ STOOL SPECIMENS

Collection

If needed, collect at least three stool samples over 10 days.
Avoid use of barium, magnesium, or oil before collection.
Other cathartics are acceptable.
Exclude urine if possible.
Waterproof or waxed-carton container is preferable.
Refrigerate if more than a half-hour delay in handling.
Feces deposited on soil may have soil-parasite contaminant.

Immediate examination

Macroscopic: Check stool for adult parasites, blood, and mucus.

Direct wet film

Dilute a drop of sample with drop of saline.
Mix on slide and place coverslip.
Dilute so that ordinary newsprint can be read through it.
Examine microscopically *unstained* first.
Adding a drop of *stain* to the edge of the coverslip may be helpful for identification (gram iodine, Lugol's solution or modified D'Antoni's iodine solution).

Delayed examination

Concentration techniques

Formalin-ether (F-E) sedimentation may be done from fresh or formalin-preserved samples.
Zinc-sulfate centrifugal flotation methods used in some laboratories.

Permanent staining

Streak thin film of sample on slide.
Mix with Gomori's trichrome stain, iron hematoxylin, or MIF (merthiolate + Lugol's iodine + formaldehyde).

Preserving

Recommended if liquid stools cannot be examined within a half hour or solid stools within 4 hours, or if sample sent by mail.
Formalin (5 or 10%) is best for subsequent concentration.
Polyvinyl alcohol (PVA) is best for subsequent staining.

▶ STOOL SPECIMENS (Cont.)

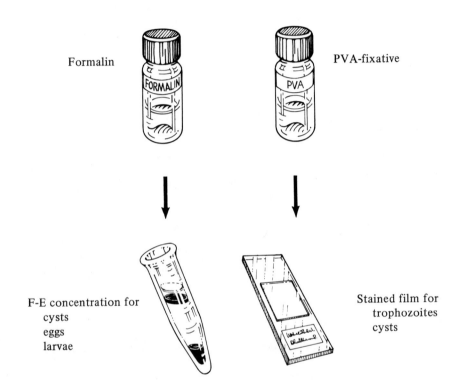

Formalin

PVA-fixative

F-E concentration for
cysts
eggs
larvae

Stained film for
trophozoites
cysts

▶ **CELLULOSE TAPE SPECIMENS FOR PINWORM OVA**
(Enterobius vermicularis)

Best taken between 10 pm and midnight, or early am before defecation.
Refrigerate if examination of specimen is delayed for more than 1 day.

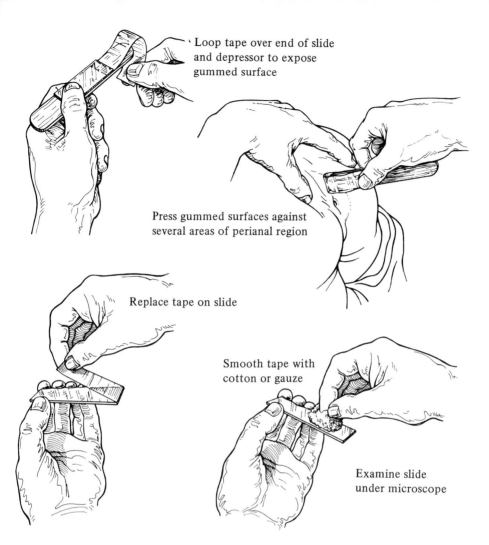

Loop tape over end of slide and depressor to expose gummed surface

Press gummed surfaces against several areas of perianal region

Replace tape on slide

Smooth tape with cotton or gauze

Examine slide under microscope

▶ SPECIMENS COLLECTED BY SIGMOIDOSCOPY FOR ENTAMOEBA HISTOLYTICA

In amebiasis, if stools are negative, material may be obtained by sigmoidoscopy. Obtain sample immediately following a normal bowel movement, or if a cathartic is given, after a lapse of 2–3 hours.

Collect the specimens with a serologic pipette rather than a cotton swab.

Aspirate (or curette) material from any visible lesion and the mucosa.

Specimens should be examined immediately.

After the direct examination, PVA fixative may be added and the preparation dried and stained.

▶ OTHER SPECIMENS

Sputum (e.g., hookworm), urine (e.g., schistosomiasis), biopsy material (e.g., trichonosis, schistosomiasis), duodenal drainage (e.g., strongyloidosis, giardiosis) may also be helpful for identifying certain intestinal parasites.

▶ **RECOGNITION OF INTESTINAL PARASITES**

Adult parasite size:

Microscopic	0.5 cm	0.5 cm–1.5 cm	1.5 cm–5 cm	50 cm

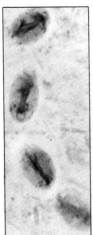
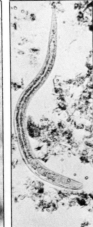
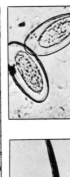
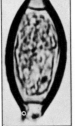

Giardia lambdia *Strongyloides stercoralis* (pinworm) *Enterobius vermicularis* (whipworm) *Trichuris trichiura* *Ascaris lumbricoides*

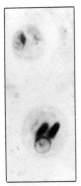
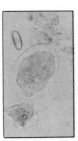
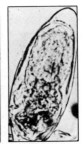

Entamoeba histolytica *Necator americanus* or *Ancylostoma duodenale* (hookworm) *Schistosoma mansoni*

SEROLOGY

Serologic tests are useful in measuring the level of disease-specific antibodies present in a patient's serum. Though they are most commonly carried out on serum, other specimens such as spinal fluid, brain tissue, and vesicular fluid may be used. Serology is extremely valuable in the diagnosis of viral, rickettsial, and fungal infections and, to a lesser extent, certain bacterial and parasitic diseases.

▶ AVAILABLE TESTS

There are a number of serologic tests available. The most commonly utilized are:
- Complement fixation tests (CF)
- Neutralizing antibody tests (N)
- Hemagglutination inhibition tests (HI)
- Fluorescent antibody tests (FA)
- Agglutination tests (Agg)

▶ REPORTING AND INTERPRETATION OF RESULTS

Serologic tests are reported as antibody titers (for example, 1:4, 1:8, 1:16, 1:32, etc.). The higher the number, the more antibodies are present. Changes in titers over time provide the most useful information. Preferably two specimens for titers are obtained: one called an *acute* specimen, collected during the first few days of the illness, and the second called a *convalescent* specimen, collected several weeks after the onset of illness. The difference between the two titers must usually be at least fourfold in order to interpret a test as indicating *recent* infection. A single, very high titer, however, may also suggest recent infection.

Bacterial diseases	Serological test for antibody[a]			
	CF	AGG	HA	ASO-ADNB-AH
Anthrax				
Bartonellosis				
Botulism			X	
Brucellosis		X		
Chancroid				
Cholera				
Conjunctivitis				
Diarrhea				
Diphtheria			X	
Dysentery (shig.)				
Food poisoning				
Glanders				
Gonococcal infection				
Klebsiella infection				
Leprosy				
Leptospirosis		X		
Listeriosis		X		
Meningitis				
Melioidosis		X		
Paratyphoid fever		X		
Pertussis				
Pinta				
Plague			X	
Pneumonia				
Rat-bite fever		X		
Relapsing fever				X
Rheumatic fever				
Salmonellosis				
Shigellosis				
Staphylococcal infection				
Streptococcal infection				X
Syphilis	(all standard tests)			
Tetanus			X	
Tuberculosis and other mycobacterial infections				
Tularemia		X		
Typhoid fever				
Yaws				

[a] CF = Complement fixation; AGG = Agglutination; HA = Hemagglutination; ASO = Anti-streptolysin-O; ADNB = Anti DNaseB; AH = Antihyaluronidase; X = available tests.

Disease syndrome	Associated agent	Serologic test [a]			
		CF	N	HI	FA
Central Nervous System					
Meningoencephalitis	Arboviruses (dengue, yellow fever, eastern equine, etc.)	Ⓧ	X	Ⓧ	
	Poliovirus	Ⓧ	X		
	Enterovirus	Ⓧ			
	Lymphocytic choriomeningitis	X	X		
	Rabies		X		Ⓧ
	Herpes simplex	Ⓧ	X		
Respiratory System					
Influenza	Influenza group	Ⓧ	X	Ⓧ	
Acute respiratory disease and pneumonia	Adenovirus group	Ⓧ	X	X	
	Parainfluenza	Ⓧ	X	X	
	Respiratory syncytial	Ⓧ	X		
	Psittacosis	Ⓧ			
	Mycoplasma pneumoniae	Ⓧ	X	X	
Vesicular Diseases					
Vesicular eruptions	Variola-Vaccinia	Ⓧ	X		X
	Chickenpox–herpes zoster	Ⓧ			X
	Herpes simplex	Ⓧ	X		
Miscellaneous					
Rocky Mountain spotted fever, typhus, etc.	Rickettsiae	Ⓧ			
Herpangina	Coxsackie A group	Ⓧ			
Pleurodynia, pericarditis, myocarditis	Coxsackie B group	Ⓧ			

Ⓧ Most commonly used tests   [a]CF = Complement fixation. N = Neutralization.
X   Alternative tests   HI = Hemagglutination inhibition.
                             FA = Fluorescent antibody.

(Continued on next page)

SEROLOGIC TESTS FOR VIRAL AND RICKETTSIAL DISEASES (Cont.)

Disease syndrome	Associated agent	Serologic test[a]			
		CF	N	HI	FA
Hand, foot, mouth syndrome	Coxsackie A16		(X)		
Mumps		(X)		X	
Measles		(X)		X	
Rubella (German measles)		X	X	(X)	X
Epidemic kerato-conjunctivitis	Adenovirus	(X)	X	X	
Lymphogranuloma venereum		(X)			
Cytomegalic inclusion disease	Cytomegalovirus	(X)			
Infectious mononucleosis		Agglutination and FA			

IMMUNODIAGNOSTIC TESTS FOR PARASITIC INFECTIONS

Parasitic diseases	Intradermal	Complement fixation	Precipitin	Agglutination	Flocculation	Hemagglutination	Latex agglutination	Fluorescent antibody	Methylene blue dye test	ELISA	RIA
Ascariasis	◎	◎	◉			◉					
Trichinosis	●	●	●		●	◉	◉			◎	◉
Toxocariasis	◎				◎	◎				◎	◎
Cysticercosis		●	●								
Echinococcosis	●	●	◉		●	●				◎	◎
Schistosomiasis	◉	◉	◉	◎	◉	◉					
Clonorchiasis	◉	◉				◎					
Paragonimiasis	◉	◉									
Filariasis	◉	◉								◎	◎
Chagas' disease	◎	◉	◎	◎				◎	◎		
Leishmaniasis	◉	◉								◎	◎
Toxoplasmosis	◉	◉		◎		◉ [a]		◉	●	◎	◎
Amebiasis		◉	◎								

◎ Under experimental investigation.
◉ Clinical usefulness limited.
● Generally accepted useful routine diagnostic test.

[a] Used for screening.

Note: Check with CDC for latest update.

SEROLOGIC TESTS FOR SYSTEMIC MYCOSES

Serologic tests are only of minor clinical importance
in the diagnosis of systemic mycoses.

Disease	CF	N	HI	FA	Agg	Other
Aspergillosis						Precipitins
Blastomycosis	X					
Candidiasis						Precipitins
Coccidioidomycosis	X				X	Precipitins
Cryptococcosis				X	X	
Histoplasmosis	X				X	

| | | | *Serologic tests* | | | |

ARTHROPODS OF MEDICAL IMPORTANCE

Arthropod ectoparasites play an important role in the transmission of plague,
typhus, tularemia, spotted fever, relapsing fever, and several other diseases
caused by bacteria, viruses, or rickettsia.

▶ IDENTIFICATION

Ticks and mites have eight legs in the nymphal and adult stages. Fleas and lice
are true insects with six legs. Fleas are very active, compressed from side to side,
with elongated legs adapted for jumping. Lice are more sluggish, flat insects,
with legs adapted for grasping hairs.

▶ **COLLECTION FOR IDENTIFICATION**

Collect ticks, mites, fleas, and lice from animal bedding, burrows, or bird nests, with fine forceps, aspirators, or applicator sticks. They may also be combed or brushed off infested animals.

Insect nets, aspirators, chloroform tubes, cyanide jars, light traps, bait traps, or fly traps are helpful. Barns, outbuildings, and the undersurfaces of bridges are preferred resting places for adults during the day. Submit all specimens unmounted.

▶ **SHIPPING FOR IDENTIFICATION**

Moist	*Dry*
In 70% alcohol	*In pill boxes between layers of tissue or lens paper (not cotton)* *DO NOT MOUNT SPECIMENS*
Ticks	Mosquitos
Mites	Flies
Fleas	True bugs
Lice	Wasps, bees
Fly maggots	Moths
Spiders	Butterflies
Mosquito larvae	Gnats
Gnats	
Bedbugs	
Ants	
Caterpillars	

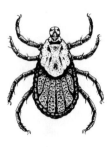

Dermacentor andersoni—
Rocky Mountain Wood Tick

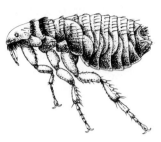

Ctenocephalides felix—
Cat Flea

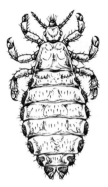

Pediculus humanus—
Human Head and Body Louse

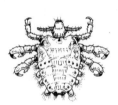

Pthirus pubis—
Human Crab Louse

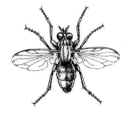

Musca domestic—
House Fly

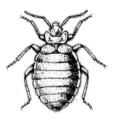

Cimex lectularius—
Bed Bug

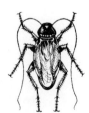

Periplaneta americana—
American Cockroach

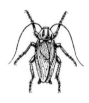

Blatella germanica—
German Cockroach

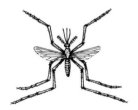

Anopheles quadrimaculatus—
Malaria Mosquito

PREPARATION AND SHIPMENT
OF MICROBIAL SPECIMENS

- Select appropriate specimens, based on clinical history and disease suspected.
- Select appropriate transport media if required (see page 192).
- Label individual specimens with name, type of specimen, and date. Type or pencil on adhesive tape (ink runs when wet).
- Include brief clinical history and indicate the etiologic agent suspected.
- Pack to prevent breakage or spillage.
    - Enclose the specimen in a 2-ml, or larger, bottle or tube of thick glass or plastic sealed with a rubber stopper. Additionally seal it by wrapping the closure with tape. *Screwcaps and ordinary corks are not recommended* for blood, serum, or other fluid specimens because of potential for leakage. Screwcaps are acceptable for agar slants or similar cultures, provided they have a resilient liner and are secured by tape. Capped jars should, in addition, be secured with a metal collar or adhesive tape. Gas-forming cultures or yeast are an exception to this rule.
    - Place the glass or plastic container in a watertight can (paint cans are suitable). Pack absorbent cotton or other suitable absorbent material around the container to absorb shock and possible leakage. Do not use particulate material. If several tubes are packed in the same can, wrap them individually in paper toweling or cotton.
    - *Note:* Never mail specimens in Petri plates or use dry ice in sealed containers.
- Mark shipments of diagnostic specimens "Perishable," "Packed in Dry Ice," "Refrigerated Biologic Material," or "Fragile," as appropriate. Label shipments containing etiologic agents (cultures, etc.).
- Time shipments to arrive during the work week, *not* just before or on a weekend or holiday.
- Statutes and regulations exist governing shipments of etiologic agents and diagnostic specimens between countries and between states within the USA. Check with the local health department before sending material.
- *Note:* If shipment is being sent to CDC, address to:

> Center for Disease Control
> Attn: Data and Specimen Handling Activity
> Bureau of Laboratories
> Atlanta, Georgia 30333

6

IMMUNIZATIONS

SCHEDULES FOR ROUTINE, ACTIVE IMMUNIZATIONS

NORMAL INFANTS AND CHILDREN

Age

2 months	DTP[a]	and	TOPV[b]
4 months	DTP	and	(TOPV optional)
6 months	DTP	and	TOPV
15 months	Measles-rubella	and	(Mumps optional)[c]
			Tuberculin test[d]
1 1/2 years	DTP	and	TOPV
4–6 years	DTP	and	TOPV
14–16 years	Td[e]		and thereafter every 10 years[f]

[a] DTP = Diptheria and tetanus toxoids combined with pertussis vaccine. Give IM.

[b] TOPV = Trivalent oral poliovirus vaccine. This recommendation is suitable for breast-fed as well as bottle-fed infants.

[c] May be given as measles-rubella or measles-mumps-rubella combined vaccines.

[d] Frequency of repeated tuberculin tests depends on risk of exposure of the child and on the prevalence of tuberculosis in the population.

[e] Td = Combined tetanus and diphtheria toxoids (adult type) for those over 6 years (contains less diphtheria antigen).

[f] For contaminated wounds, a booster dose should be given at time of injury if more than 5 years have elapsed since the last dose.

Note: Measles vaccine may be given simultaneously with the tuberculin (usually tine) test in geographic areas where the risk of having tuberculosis is low, or in individual children who may not return for follow-up visits. Temporary interruptions do not affect the schedule (continue at the point where immunizations were stopped). Dosages may vary with manufacturer. Most vaccines must be stored to protect from heat and light.

PRIMARY IMMUNIZATION FOR CHILDREN NOT IMMUNIZED IN INFANCY [a]

15 months through 5 years of age

First visit	DTP, TOPV, tuberculin test
1 month later	Measles, rubella (mumps optional)
2 months later	DTP, TOPV
4 months later	DTP, (TOPV optional)
6–12 months later or at preschool	DTP, TOPV
Age, 14–16 years	Td; thereafter every 10 years

6 years of age and over

Same as above but use Td in place of DTP.

[a] Physicians may choose to alter the sequence of these schedules if specific infections are prevalent at the time.

CONTRAINDICATIONS TO VACCINATION

Condition	Comments
Pregnancy	Mumps, measles, rubella contraindicated. Others should be used only if urgently required (see page 220).
Eczema in recipient or family member.	Smallpox inoculation contraindicated.
Acute severe febrile illness [a]	All vaccines should be withheld until illness is over.
Immunosuppressive therapy (steroids, irradication, antimetabolites, alkylating agents; leukemia, lymphoma, or other generalized malignancy; cellular immunodeficiencies).	Live virus vaccines are contraindicated since they may cause overwhelming infections.
Sensitivity or allergy to certain animal proteins.	Select the live virus vaccines that are grown in preparations to which the person is not sensitive. If sensitivity suspected, administer in appropriate clinical setting.
Convulsion reaction to DTP vaccine	Complete the vaccination program with DT (omit pertussis vaccine) if patient is 6 years old or under or Td if patient is over 6 years old. (Td contains less diphtheria toxoid than DT).

[a] Minor illnesses such as a cold not associated with fever should *not* delay vaccination.

GUIDE TO USE OF IMMUNIZING AGENTS FOR SPECIAL HIGH-RISK SITUATIONS

Disease	Immunizing Agent	For high-risk groups	Dose and schedule	Administration route	Boosters if exposure persists
Cholera	Active: Bacterial antigen	All ages (see page 22)	2 doses (age dependent) 1 month apart	Subcut or IM	Every 6 months
Diphtheria	Active: Toxoid	Not under 2 months (see page 218 for routine immunizations)	0.5 ml, 3 doses (see page 28).	IM	Every 10 years
	Passive: Antitoxin	All ages (see page 28)			None
Hepatitis, type A	Passive: Immune serum globulin (ISG)	All ages (see page 44)	Variable (see page 44)	IM	Every 6 months
Hepatitis, type B	Passive: Immune serum globulin (ISG)	All ages (see page 46)	2 doses 1 month apart 0.12 ml/kg	IM	None
	Hepatitis B immune globulin (HBIG)		0.06 ml/kg	IM	None
Influenza	Active: Inactivated virus	*Not* under 3 months of age (see page 54)	Dose and schedule age-dependent (see page 54)	Subcut	Seasonally
Measles (rubeola)	Active: Live virus	(See page 218 for routine immunizations)	Single dose	IM	None
	Passive: Immune serum globulin (ISG)	All ages (see page 60)	0.25 mg/kg immediately after exposure	IM	None

Disease	Agent	Indication	Dosage	Route	Booster
Mumps	Active: Live virus	(See page 218 for routine immunizations)		IM	None
	Passive: ISG		Single dose 20–40 ml	IM or IV	None
Pertussis	Active: Bacterial antigen		3 doses, 0.5 ml (see page 70)	IM	None over age 6
	Passive: ISG			IM	None
Plague	Active: Bacterial antigen		3 doses (age dependent) spaced 1 month apart	IM	Every 6–12 months x 2, then every 1–2 years
Pneumococcal infections	Active: Bacterial antigen	*Not* under 2 years of age (see page 74)	Single dose (check circular)	Subcut or IM	None, but experience limited to 2-year follow up
Polio	Active: Live virus	(See page 218 for routine immunizations)	3 doses, 2 drops (see page 76)	Oral	Usually none
Rabies	Active: Killed virus vaccine (DEV)	Pre and postexposure (see page 78)	1 ml schedule depends on indication	Subcut	Every 1–3 years
	Passive: Human rabies immune globulin (HRIG)	All ages (see page 78)	Single dose (1/2 IM, 1/2 local) 20 IU/kg	IM and local	None
	Antirabies serum, equine (ARS)	All ages (see page 78)	40 IU/kg	IM and local	None

(Continued on next page)

GUIDE TO USE OF IMMUNIZING AGENTS FOR SPECIAL HIGH-RISK SITUATIONS (Cont.)

Disease	Immunizing agent	For high-risk groups	Dose and schedule	Administration route	Boosters if exposure persists
Rubella	Active: Live virus	(See page 218 for routine immunization)	Once	IM	None
	Passive: Standard immune serum globulin	Limited value		IM	None
Smallpox	Active: Live vaccinia virus	All ages, but if possible defer until second year of life (see page 138)	1 inoculation: multiple pressure through 1 drop vaccine over deltoid. Blot excess. No dressing.	Skin puncture	Every 3 years
	Passive: Vaccinia immune globulin (human, VIG)	For those with severe "vaccinia" infections or with severe skin disease and exposed to vaccinia (check with CDC)	Usually 0.3 ml/kg	IM	Check with CDC or health department
Tetanus	Active: Toxoid	(See page 218 for routine immunization) (See page 102)	3 doses, 0.5 ml (see page 218)	IM	Every 10 years after initial series
	Passive: Tetanus immune globulin (TIG, human)			IM	None

Tuberculosis	Active: BCG	All ages (see page 108)	Single dose 0.05 ml for newborns, 0.1 ml for others	Intracutaneous or multiple puncture	None
Typhoid	Active: Bacterial antigen	*Not* under 6 months of age (see page 110)	2 doses of 0.5 cc (0.25 cc if under 10 years old) 3 weeks apart	Subcut	Every 3 years
Typhus	Active: Bacterial antigen	(See page 134)	2 doses 4 weeks apart (check circular)	Subcut or IM	Every 6–12 months
Varicella	Passive: Zoster immune globulin (ZIG, human)	(See page 112)	Single dose	IM	None
Yellow fever	Active: Live attenuated virus	(See page 114)	Single dose	Subcut or IM	Every 10 years

GUIDELINES FOR IMMUNIZATION DURING PREGNANCY

Pregnant women should avoid being immunized whenever possible. The following is a guide to help decide if immunization is warranted.

1. *Confirm* the pregnancy.

2. *Prevent exposure* by stressing sanitary precautions (against hepatitis, typhoid, and cholera) and advising against travel to areas endemic for plague, yellow fever, or smallpox. Advise limiting contact with people who may be sick with locally endemic or epidemic diseases like measles, rubella, or influenza.

3. *Determine the susceptibility* of the patient to the vaccine—preventable disease by history of illnesses and vaccinations. Use serology whenever indicated (e.g., for rubella, an HI antibody titer of less than 1:8 confirms susceptibility to infection and need for vaccination immediately postpartum).

4. *Determine the degree of exposure.* Some diseases are extremely infectious (rubella, measles, mumps, chickenpox, and influenza) whereas others are much less so (diphtheria, typhoid fever, and hepatitis).

5. *Determine the risk of serious illness:*
   - For the pregnant woman (see table).
   - For the fetus or newborn (see table).

6. *Not all vaccines* are completely effective. Cholera, typhoid, and influenza vaccines only offer poor or short-term immunity. Other vaccines, though perhaps more than 90% effective, must be administered early enough after exposure to be able to stimulate immunity or alter the course of the disease.

7. *Determine the risk of vaccination* for the fetus (see table).

The table on pages 227 and 228 is a guide to help determine the risks involved.

GUIDE TO IMMUNIZATION DURING PREGNANCY

Disease	Does pregnancy increase the severity of the disease in women?	What is the risk of the disease for the fetus or newborn	Vaccine type	Risk from vaccine to fetus	Should the pregnant woman be vaccinated?
Tetanus Diphtheria	No	Neonatal tetanus has 60% mortality	Toxoids [a] (combined)	NC [b]	Yes, if primary series lacking, or no booster in 10 years
Polio	Possibly	Possible fetal damage and 50% mortality in newborn	Live virus	NC	Only in epidemic situations
Mumps	No	?	Live virus	NC	Never
Measles	No	Increased abortion rate	Live virus	NC	Never—consider use of gamma globulin
Rubella	No	High abortion rate and congenital rubella syndrome	Live virus	NC	Never—even though risk highest in first trimester
Influenza	Possibly	Possible increased abortion rate	Inactivated virus	NC	Only if woman has *serious* cardiac, pulmonary, or metabolic disease
Typhoid	No	?	Killed bacteria	NC	Only if exposure is close and continued

(Continued on next page)

225

GUIDE TO IMMUNIZATION DURING PREGNANCY (Cont.)

Disease	Does pregnancy increase the severity of the disease in women?	What is the risk of the disease for the fetus or newborn	Vaccine type	Risk from vaccine to fetus	Should the pregnant woman be vaccinated?
Smallpox	Yes	Possible increased abortion rate	Live virus	Congenital vaccinia rare	Only in cases of probable exposure
Yellow fever	No	?	Live virus	?	Only in cases of unavoidable exposure—better to postpone travel
Cholera	No	?	Killed bacteria	?	Only to meet international travel requirements
Plague	No	?	Killed bacteria	None reported	Only in cases of extreme exposure
Rabies	No (almost 100% fatal)	Determined by outcome of mother's illness	Killed virus	?	Yes, management not to be altered due to pregnancy
Hepatitis-A	No	Transmission to fetus possible neonatal hepatitis	Immune globulin	None reported	Yes, management not to be altered due to pregnancy
Varicella	No	Increased risk of severe disease	Immune globulin	None reported	Only if known susceptible and exposed

[a]Toxoids are preparations of chemically altered bacterial exotoxins.   [b]None confirmed, but cases reported.

Adapted from American College of Obstetricians and Gynecologists, *Technical Bulletin*, No. 20, March 1973.

IMMUNIZATIONS FOR INTERNATIONAL TRAVEL

▶ VACCINATION CERTIFICATE REQUIREMENTS

Under the International Health Regulations adopted by WHO, a country may, under certain conditions, require *International Certificates of Vaccination* against:

Type	Doses	Comments
Cholera	1	Certificate valid for 6 months beginning 6 days after 1 injection of vaccine or on the date of revaccination if within 6 months of first injection.
Smallpox	1	Certificate valid for 3 years beginning 8 days after successful primary vaccination or on the date of revaccination.
Yellow fever	1	Certificate valid for 10 years beginning 10 days after primary vaccination or on the date of revaccination if within 10 years of first injection.

▶ DETERMINATION OF REQUIREMENTS

List the traveler's itinerary in the sequence in which the countries will be visited. Consider the length of stay in each country. For the purpose of the International Health Regulations, the incubation periods of the *quarantinable diseases* are:

Cholera	5 days	Smallpox	14 days
Plague	6 days	Yellow fever	6 days

Check the current weekly Blue Sheet* to determine if any country on the itinerary is currently infected with cholera, smallpox, or yellow fever. This is essential because some countries require vaccination only if a traveler arrives from an infected area.

---

*The Bureau of Epidemiology, CDC, distributes a weekly "Blue Sheet" (countries with areas infected with quarantinable diseases) that shows which countries are currently reporting these diseases.

Travelers should be advised to contact their local health department, physician, or private or public agency that advises international travelers at least 2 weeks prior to departure to obtain current information on countries to be visited.

▶ DETERMINATION OF REQUIREMENTS (Cont.)

Use the Vaccination Certificate Requirements section of a booklet entitled "Health Information for International Traveler," printed and distributed by CDC, to determine the vaccinations required by each country.

▶ EXEMPTION FROM VACCINATION

Age: Some countries do not require International Certificates of Vaccination for infants under 13 months of age.

Medical grounds: If a physician thinks that vaccination should not be performed on medical grounds, the traveler should be given a signed, dated statement of these reasons on the physician's letterhead stationery.

There are no other acceptable reasons for exemption from vaccination.

It is best to check with the embassy or local consulate general office of the country in question about such situations before traveling.

▶ PERSONS AUTHORIZED TO VACCINATE, TO SIGN, AND TO VALIDATE CERTIFICATES

The certificates must be signed by a licensed physician or by a person under his supervision whom he has designated to sign them. *A signature stamp is not acceptable.*

Vaccinations may be given under the supervision of any licensed physician. Validation of the certificate can be obtained at many health departments, or from vaccinating physicians who possess a "uniform stamp." Yellow fever vaccinations must be given at an officially designated yellow fever center, and the certificate must be validated by the same center. Failure to secure validation may cause a traveler to be revaccinated or quarantined.

▶ UNVACCINATED PERSONS

Travelers who do not have the required vaccinations may be denied entry, or may be subject to vaccination, medical follow-up, and/or isolation upon entering a country.

▶ REQUIREMENTS FOR UNITED STATES TRAVELERS

To Europe: No vaccinations.

To Canada and Mexico: No vaccinations.

▶ MISCELLANEOUS PREEXPOSURE VACCINATIONS AND PROPHYLAXES

Plague, rabies, TB (BCG), typhoid, and typhus vaccines are never required, and usually not recommended for short-term (less than 3 month) recreation travelers who use ordinary tourist routes.

Immune serum globulin (ISG) for hepatitis prevention is similarly rarely recommended.

Malaria and *E. coli* chemoprophylaxis may be recommended depending on time and place. Check with the health department.

7

INFECTIOUS DISEASE CONTROL MEASURES

CONTENTS

Patient Isolation Techniques
Selected Measures To Limit Spread of
 Infectious Diseases
Antiseptics and Disinfectants
Reporting of Infectious Diseases
Preventing Infections Among Employees
Outbreak Investigation

PATIENT ISOLATION TECHNIQUES

The costs of isolating patients must always be considered. They include personnel time, money for disposables, equipment or room availability, and psychological impact on patient.

Compromises in technique are frequently required due to limited resources and patient loads. Isolation should be terminated as soon as possible. Isolation door signs are available from CDC.

▶ STRICT ISOLATION

Private room—necessary. Door must be kept closed, specially ventilated room preferred.
Gowns—must be worn by all persons entering room.
Masks—must be worn by all persons entering room.
Hands—must be washed after contact with patient or dressing, and upon leaving the room.
Gloves—must be worn by all persons having contact with patient or dressing.
Articles—special precautions necessary for instruments, dressings, linen, and dishes.

Diseases requiring strict isolation

Anthrax, inhalation*
Burns, extensive, infected with
　Staphylococcus aureus or
　group A streptococcus
Diphtheria
Eczema vaccinatum
Melioidosis, pulmonary, or
　extrapulmonary with draining
　sinuses
Neonatal vesicular disease (herpes
　simplex)

Plague*
Rabies
Congenital rubella syndrome
Smallpox*
Staphylococcal enterocolitis
Staphylococcal pneumonia
Streptococcal pneumonia
Vaccinia, generalized and progressive

▶ RESPIRATORY ISOLATION
(Droplet nuclei)

Private room—necessary. Door must be kept closed, specially ventilated room preferred.
Masks—must be worn by all persons entering room and by patient if possible.

*Specially ventilated room mandatory.

▶ RESPIRATORY ISOLATION (Cont.)

Diseases requiring respiratory isolation*

Chickenpox	Pertussis (whooping cough)
Herpes zoster	Rubella (German measles)
Measles (rubeola)	Tuberculosis, pulmonary—
Meningococcal meningitis	sputum-positive (or suspect)
Meningococcemia	Venezuelan equine
Mumps	encephalomyelitis

▶ WOUND AND SKIN PRECAUTIONS

Private room—desirable (two-bed room permissible).

Gowns—must be worn by all persons having direct contact with patient or dressings.

Masks—not necessary except during dressing changes.

Hands—must be washed after contact with patient or dressings, and on leaving room.

Gloves—must be worn by all persons having direct contact with patient or dressings.

Articles—special precautions necessary for instruments, dressings, and linen.

Diseases requiring wound and skin precautions

Burns, (infected)	Streptococcal skin infection
Gas gangrene	Wound infection, extensive
Impetigo	
Staphylococcal skin and wound infections	

▶ ENTERIC PRECAUTIONS

Private room—necessary for children. Private room desirable for infants and adults. Two-bed room permissible.

Gowns—must be worn by all persons having direct contact with patient.

Hands—must be washed after contact with patient.

Gloves—must be worn by all persons having direct contact with patient or with articles contaminated with fecal material.

Articles—special precautions necessary for linen, dishes, and articles contaminated with urine and/or feces.

Diseases requiring enteric precautions

Cholera	Salmonellosis (including typhoid fever)
Enteropathogenic *E. coli,* gastroenteritis	Shigellosis
Hepatitis, viral	Viral gastroenteritis

*Acute, active, untreated cases should be in specially ventilated isolation rooms.

▶ PROTECTIVE ISOLATION

Private room—necessary. Door must be kept closed.
Gowns—must be worn by all persons entering room.
Masks—must be worn by all persons entering room.
Hands—must be washed before direct contact with patient.
Gloves—must be worn by all persons having direct contact with patient.

Conditions that may require protective isolation

Agranulocytosis or severe leukopenia.
Severe and extensive, noninfected vasicular, bullous, or eczematous dermatitis.
Extensive noninfected burns, until application of protective topical therapy (Sulfamylon or silver nitrate).
Certain patients receiving immunosuppressive therapy.
Certain patients with lymphomas and leukemia.

GUIDE TO HOSPITAL ISOLATION FOR SOME DISEASES TRANSMITTED BY RESPIRATORY SECRETIONS

Diseases	Isolation of patient	Wear mask	Wear clean gown	Wear gloves	Duration of isolation
Diphtheria [a]	S	Yes	Yes	No	(b)
Chickenpox, measles, mumps, and pertussis [a]	R	Yes	Yes	No	See page 233
Staphylococcal respiratory diseases	S	Yes	Yes	For direct contact	DI
Hemolytic streptococcal respiratory diseases	S	Yes	Yes	For direct contact	First day of treatment
Influenza and other viral respiratory diseases	None	No	No	No	None
Meningococcal meningitis	R	No	Yes	No	First day of treatment
Tuberculosis, sputum positive	R	Yes	No	No	Until sputum negative

[a] Admit visitors only if immune.
[b] Until two cultures taken at least 24 hours apart are negative. Culture nose and throat after cessation of therapy.

GUIDE TO HOSPITAL ISOLATION FOR DISEASES TRANSMITTED BY ENTERAL ROUTE OR DIRECT CONTACT

Diseases	Isolation of patient	Wear mask	Wear clean gown	Wear gloves	Duration of isolation
Transmitted by enteral route					
Acute diarrheal diseases	E	No	For direct contact	For direct contact	DI
Hepatitis A	E	No	Yes	No	2 weeks from onset
Transmitted by direct contact					
Primary or secondary syphilis	Lesion contact precautions	No	No	First day of treatment	First day of treatment
Gonorrhea, chancroid, granuloma inguinale, lymphogranuloma venereum	No	No	No	Before treatment	None
Wound infections, pyoderma	Lesion contact precautions	No	For direct contact	For direct contact	DI

Note: In all cases, provision should be made for sanitary disposal of contaminated articles. All who contact the isolation area should wash hands upon leaving.

(1) Until two cultures taken at least 24 hours apart are negative. Culture nose and throat after cessation of therapy. DI = Duration of illness; R = Respiratory precautions; S = Strict isolation; E = Enteric precautions.

SELECTED MEASURES TO LIMIT SPREAD
OF INFECTIOUS DISEASES
IN HOSPITAL, CLINIC, OR HOME

Many of the measures listed will have to be modified depending on the circumstances, and may be adapted for hospital, clinic, or home use.

▶ HANDWASHING

Conscientious handwashing is an important step in the control of communicable disease. Careful attention to washing with soap and water and/or antibacterial solutions should be carried out when: hands are obviously soiled, between handling of each patient, before contact with patient's face or mouth, before eating, after use of the toilet, after blowing or wiping the nose, after any contact with the isolation area, after handling excretion (feces, urine, etc.) or secretions (wounds, skin infection, etc.), on completion of patient care.

▶ CLEANSING THERMOMETERS

- Water-soluble lubricants should be used on rectal thermometers.
- Wash in soap and water, then disinfect with a solution of 70–90% ethyl or isopropyl alcohol with 0.2% iodine. Cover the thermometer completely.
- Change solution and wash container twice weekly with soap and water.

▶ MASKING

- Check isolation techniques (see page 232) for indications for use.
- Masks should always cover both nose and mouth.
- Masks are less effective when damp.
- Discard used masks in appropriate receptacles.

▶ GOWNS AND APRONS

- Check isolation techniques for indications for use.
- Gowns are most useful when: giving direct patient care, medications, or feeding the patient; making the bed; doing housekeeping duties in an isolation unit; giving treatments and changing wound dressings.
- If discarding after one use is impractical, a reuse technique should be devised.

▶ CARING FOR LINEN

- Use linen bag or pillow case for collecting linen.
- Remove blood, feces, and other soil from linen, including diapers, before laundering.
- Use double-bag technique if it is necessary to transport contaminated linen.
- Dispose of diapers in can with inside liner. Use disposable diapers when possible.

▶ **EATING UTENSILS**

- In the home, wash eating utensils separately with soap and hot running water, rinse and air dry.
- Keep utensils covered and separate until the infectious period is over.
- Boil utensils for 15 minutes before returning them to general family use.
- When feasible use disposable plates and utensils. A second washing is advisable in an automatic dishwasher, if available.

▶ **SERVING FOOD**

- Gown or apron may be useful (check isolation techniques).
- If necessary, help patient with handwashing.
- Transfer meal to infectious patient's tray at doorway.
- Discard leftover solid food and disposable utensils into a paper bag with shredded paper, wrap securely, and dispose with regular garbage.
- Throw liquids, soft and pulpy food into toilet.
- Clean tray and wash nondisposable utensils according to isolation procedure established for the situation.

▶ **DRESSING WOUNDS OF PATIENTS AT HOME**

- Wash hands before and after procedure.
- Explain the procedure to patient and family to help allay apprehensions.
- Disposable (or home) equipment should be used whenever possible.
- Minimize talking and movement while wound is exposed, to prevent dispersal of pathogens into and from wound.
- Sterilize equipment in oven using 350F for 1 hour or use pressure cooker at 121C for 15 minutes. Equipment requiring disinfection can be boiled for 15 minutes (*not sterile*).
- Carefully close and wrap paper bag of disposables in several thicknesses of newspaper, fastening securely and labeling "contaminated" and dispose. Incineration or autoclaving is ideal.
- Wash all used instruments and basins in soap and water and boil for 15 minutes (*not sterile*).
- If apron or gown is left in home, remove and place contaminated side folded in, inside paper bag for family to launder.

▶ **ADMINISTERING MEDICATIONS AND TREATMENTS**

- Equipment for repeated treatment should be cleaned and kept in patient's room.
- Sterilize or disinfect equipment before returning to general use.
- Disposables.

▶ **DISPOSAL OF BODY DISCHARGES**

- Make receptacles conveniently accessible to the patient.
- Cover containers to prevent spillage, odors, and contamination of environment and access by insects.

▶ DISPOSAL OF BODY DISCHARGES (Cont.)

- Use containers impermeable to liquid contents.
- Remove feces, urine, and vomitus from the patient's room and dispose of immediately in toilet. If flush toilet is not available, disinfect by: placing excreta (solids broken up) into a 2-quart container of a 5% solution (1-1/2 oz to 1 quart of water) of creosol-type disinfectant for 1 hour.

▶ CLEANING

- Clean surfaces prior to disinfection. Soil that is present may neutralize the disinfectant. Disinfectants by definition do not destroy all of the microorganisms, but do reduce the number present if used correctly.
- Wet mops, sponges, and cloths often harbor microorganisms. Store in dry conditions and clean after each day used.
- Select cleaning compounds carefully. Many are toxic. Compounds formulated for floor cleaning may be toxic for direct contact (e.g., on walls).
- Keep disinfectants in contact with surfaces for 10 minutes if possible.

▶ DISINFECTION—Concurrent

This is accomplished through:

- Immediate and proper discard of used disposable articles.
- Prompt cleaning of all washable, reusable items (see above).

▶ DISINFECTION—Terminal

To render the personal effects and immediate environment of the patient free from infective organisms, use the same methods as above, in addition to the following:

- Use of complete protective clothing during cleaning by workers.
- All receptacles (drainage bottles, urinals, bedpans, flowmeter jars, thermometer holders, etc.) should be emptied and wrapped.
- All disposable items should be discarded in a wastebasket lined with an impermeable plastic bag.
- All equipment should be washed with a germicidal detergent solution.
- All floors should be wet-vacuumed. If wet-vacuuming equipment is not available, floors should be mopped with a germicidal detergent solution using the double-bucket technique.
- Grossly soiled areas on walls should be washed with a germicidal detergent solution.

▶ STERILIZATION

This can be accomplished with heat, chemicals, or radiation. Small items can be sterilized in the home with 15 minutes in a pressure cooker.

Dry heat is useful for sterilizing dressings for home use. No package should be thicker than 6 inches. Bake packages 1 hour at 350F. Leave oven door slightly ajar to prevent scorching.

Refer to the table on page 240 for disinfection and sterilization of items.

▶ LAUNDERING PROCEDURES

- Water temperature above 160F (71C) for 25 minutes will kill practically all microorganisms except spores; such temperatures are recommended for use with all except delicate fabrics. Drying and ironing substantially reduce the levels of microbial contamination.

- *Colorfast cotton, linen, rayon, nylon, dacron, or orlon* can be washed in hot water in a washing machine with 1 cup of household bleach (5.25% sodium hypochlorite) added to the wash water and laundry detergent, *or* they can be washed by hand after soaking at least 10 minutes in hot water to which laundry detergent and 1 oz (2 tablespoons) of household bleach per gallon of water have been added). *White cotton* can be boiled for 10 minutes in water and then washed by the usual method or by methods outlined above.

- *Silk, wool, unfast colors (or any other fabric, if the aforementioned methods do not apply)* can be washed in warm water in a home washing machine with Lysol or other phenolic household disinfectant added to the wash water and laundry detergent, to make a final concentration of about 400 ppm of phenol. For Lysol or other products with approximately 5% phenols, add 1 cup of product to the washing machine (change quantity in inverse proportion to concentration of phenols if significantly different from 5%). After washing and rinsing, these clothes should be washed without phenols and rinsed a second time to remove all possible toxic residues of phenols. *Or* wash by hand with phenols in warm water; add 2 tablespoons (1 oz) of approximately 5% phenolic household disinfectant per gallon of warm water to the laundry detergent, and rinse thoroughly at least three times after washing.

ANTISEPTICS AND DISINFECTANTS

Chemical group	Trade product	Active antimicrobial(s)
Phenolic compounds	Lysol Pheno-Cen Ves-Phene Staphene	Orthophenyl phenolics (and other substituted phenolics)
Bisphenolic compounds	pHisoHex Gamophen	Hexachlorophene
Mercurial preparations	Merthiolate Mercresin Nylmerate	Thimerosal Orthohydroxyphenyl- mercuric chloride Phenylmercuric acetate
Iodine preparations	Betadine Wescodyne Ioprep Prepodyne	Povidone-iodine Iodine complex Iodine complex Iodine complex
Chlorine preparation	Clorox	Sodium hypochloride
Cationic quaternary ammonium compounds (quats)	Zephiran Roccal Ceepryn	Benzalkonium chloride Benzalkonium chloride Cetylpyridinium chloride

RECOMMENDATIONS FOR CHEMICAL DISINFECTION AND STERILIZATION

Objects	Chemical disinfection					
	Low level: (vegetative bacteria and fungi and influenza viruses are killed)		Intermediate level: (low-level organisms plus the tubercle bacillus and enteroviruses are killed)		High level: (low- and intermediate-level organisms plus bacterial and highly resistant fungal spores and probably hepatitis viruses are killed)	
	Agent	Duration (in minutes)	Agent	Duration (in minutes)	Agent	Duration (in hours)
Smooth, hard-surfaced objects[b]	Ethyl or isopropyl alcohol (70–90%)[a]	10	Ethyl alcohol (70–90%)	15	Formaldehyde (8%) + alcohol (70%) solution[a]	1–2
	Formaldehyde (8%) + alcohol (70%) solution[a]	5	Formaldehyde (8%) + alcohol (70%) solution[a]	10	Ethylene oxide gas	3–12[d]
	Quaternary ammonium solutions (1 : 500 aq.)[a]	10	Iodophor–500 ppm available iodine[a]	20	Aqueous formalin (20%)	12
	Iodophor—100 ppm available iodine[a]	10	Phenolic solutions (2% aq.)[a]	10	Activated glutaraldehyde (2% aq.) Cidex	10
	Phenolic solutions (1% aq.)[a]	10	Aqueous formalin (20%)	15		
	Aqueous formalin (20%)	5	Activated glutaraldehyde (2% aq.) Cidex	15		
	Activated glutaraldehyde (2% aq.) Cidex	5				
Rubber tubing and catheters[b]	Quaternary ammonium solutions (1 : 500 aq.)[a]	10	Iodophor—500 ppm available iodine[a]	20	Ethylene oxide gas	3–12[d]

[a] 0.2% sodium nitrite should be present in alcohols, formalin, formaldehyde-alcohol, quaternary ammonium, and iodophor solutions to prevent corrosion; and 0.5% sodium bicarbonate should be present in phenolic solutions to prevent corrosion.
[b] Be certain tubing is completely filled.
[c] Thermometers must be thoroughly wiped, preferably with soap and water, before disinfection or sterilization. Alcohol-iodine solutions will remove markings on poor-grade thermometers.
[d] Depending upon procedure used; more rapidly cidal for microorganisms killed with low-level and intermediate-level disinfection.
[e] Must first be cleansed, grossly free of organic soil.

(Continued on next page)

RECOMMENDATIONS FOR CHEMICAL DISINFECTION AND STERILIZATION (Cont.)

	Chemical disinfection				
Objects	Low level: (vegetative bacteria and fungi and influenza viruses are killed)		Intermediate level: (low-level organisms plus the tubercle bacillus and enteroviruses are killed)		High level: (low- and intermediate-level organisms plus bacterial and highly resistant fungal spores and probably hepatitis viruses are killed)
	Agent	Duration (in minutes)	Agent	Duration (in minutes)	Agent	Duration (in hours)
Rubber tubing and catheters[b] (Cont.)	Iodophor–100 ppm available iodine[a]	10	Phenolic solutions (2% aq.)[a]	20		
	Phenolic solutions (1% aq.)[a]	5	Activated glutaraldehyde (2% aq.) Cidex	15		
Polyethylene tubing and catheters[b]	Ethyl or isopropyl alcohol (70–90%)[a]	10	Ethyl alcohol (70–90%)	15	Formaldehyde (8%) + alcohol (70%) solution[a]	12
	Quaternary ammonium solutions (1 : 500 aq.)[a]	10	Iodophor–500 ppm available iodine[a]	20	Ethylene oxide gas	3–12[d]
	Iodophor–100 ppm available iodine[a]	10	Phenolic solutions (2% aq.)[a]	20	Aqueous formalin (20%)	12
	Phenolic solutions (1% aq.)[a]	10	Activated glutaraldehyde (2% aq.) Cidex	15	Activated glutaraldehyde (2% aq.) Cidex	10
Lensed instruments	Quaternary ammonium solutions (1 : 500 aq.)[a]	10	Aqueous formalin (20%)	15	Ethylene oxide gas	3–12[d]
	Iodophor–100 ppm available iodine[a]	10	Activated glutaraldehyde (2% aq.) Cidex	15	Aqueous formalin (20%)	12
	Phenolic solutions (1% aq.)[a]	10			Activated glutaraldehyde (2% aq.) Cidex	10
Thermometers[c] **(glass)**	Ethyl or isopropyl alcohol (70–90%)[a] + 0.2% iodine	10	Ethyl or isopropyl alcohol (70–90%)[a] + 0.2% iodine	15	Formaldehyde (8%) + alcohol (70%) solution[a]	12
					Ethylene oxide gas (cold cycle only)	3–12[d]
					Aqueous formalin (20%)	12

Object		Min		Min		Min
Thermometers[c] (glass) (Cont.)					Activated glutaraldehyde (2% aq.) Cidex	10
Hinged instruments[e]	Ethyl or isopropyl alcohol (70–90%)[a]	15	Ethyl alcohol (70–90%)	20	Ethylene oxide gas	3–12[d]
	Formaldehyde (8%) + alcohol (70%) solution[a]	10	Formaldehyde (8%) + alcohol (70%) solution[a]	15	Aqueous formalin (20%)	12
	Quaternary ammonium solutions (1 : 500 aq.)[a]	20	Iodophor—500ppm available iodine[a]	30	Activated glutaraldehyde (2% aq.) Cidex	10
	Iodophor—100 ppm available iodine[a]	20	Phenolic solutions (2% aq.)[a]	30		
	Phenolic solutions (1% aq.)[a]	15	Aqueous formalin (20%)	20		
	Aqueous formalin (20%)	10	Activated glutaraldehyde (2% aq.) Cidex	20		
	Activated glutaraldehyde (2% aq.) Cidex	10				
Inhalation and anesthesia equipment	Ethyl or isopropyl alcohol (70–90%)[a]	15	Ethyl alcohol (70–90%)	20	Ethylene oxide gas	3–12[d]
	Quaternary ammonium solutions (1 : 500 aq.)[a]	20	Activated glutaraldehyde (2% aq.) Cidex	20	Activated glutaraldehyde (2% aq.) Cidex	10
	Activated glutaraldehyde (2% aq.) Cidex	5				
Floors, furniture, walls, etc.	Quaternary ammonium solutions (1 : 500 aq.)[a]		Iodophor—500 ppm available iodine[a]		None	
	Iodophor—100 ppm available iodine[a]		Phenolic solutions (2% aq.)[a]			
	Phenolic solutions (1% aq.)[a]		Sodium hypochlorite (1%)			
	Sodium hypochlorite (2000 ppm)					

[a]0.2% sodium nitrite should be present in alcohols, formalin, formaldehyde-alcohol, quaternary ammonium, and iodophor solutions to prevent corrosion; and 0.5% sodium bicarbonate should be present in phenolic solutions to prevent corrosion.   [b]Be certain tubing is completely filled.

[c]Thermometers must be thoroughly wiped, preferably with soap and water, before disinfection or sterilization. Alcohol-iodine solutions will remove markings on poor-grade thermometers.

[d]Depending upon procedure used; more rapidly cidal for microorganisms killed with low-level and intermediate-level disinfection.

[e]Must first be cleansed, grossly free of organic soil.

REPORTING INFECTIOUS DISEASES

Regulations governing the reporting of infectious diseases are state- and country-specific. Below are general recommendations adapted from those used in the states of California and Washington. They should serve as general guidelines to be modified according to the specific regulations governing your area of practice. Check with your local health department for regulations and reporting forms. Any health personnel knowing of a case or outbreak should make a report to the local health department.

▶ **REPORTABLE DISEASES**

Amebiasis*
Anthrax*
Botulism
Brucellosis (undulant fever)
Chancroid*
Cholera
Coccidioidomycosis*
Conjunctivitis, acute infections of the
    newborn (gonorrheal ophthalmia,
    ophthalmia neonatorum, and babies'
    sore eyes in the first 21 days of life)*
Dengue
Diarrhea of the newborn
Diphtheria
Disorders characterized by lapses of
    consciousness†
Dysentery, bacillary (see shigella
    infections)
Encephalitis, viral
Fever of unknown etiology†
Food poisoning (other than botulism)
Gastroenteritis, epidemic†
German measles (rubella)*
Gonococcal infections*
Granuloma inguinale*
Hepatitis A
Hepatitis B
Impetigo†
Infectious mononucleosis†
Influenza†
Keratoconjunctivitis, epi.†
Legionnaires' disease
Leprosy (Hansen's disease)
Leptospirosis (including Weil's disease)
Lymphocytic choriomeningitis†
Lymphogranuloma venereum
    (lymphogranuloma inguinale)*

Malaria
Measles (rubeola)*
Meningitis, viral
Meningococcal infections
Mumps*
Paratyphoid fever, A, B, and C
    (see salmonella infections)
Pertussis (whooping cough)*
Plague
Pneumonia, infectious†
Poliomyelitis, paralytic
Psittacosis
Q fever
Rabies, human or animal
Relapsing fever
Rheumatic fever, acute*
Ringworm
Rocky Mountain spotted fever
Salmonella, infectious (exclusive of
    typhoid fever)*
Scarlet fever*
Shigella infections*
Smallpox (variola)
Streptococcal infections, hemolytic
    (including scarlet fever, and
    streptococcal sore throat)*
Syphilis
Tetanus
Trachoma*
Trichinosis
Tuberculosis
Tularemia
Typhoid fever, cases and carriers
Typhus fever
Viral exanthem in pregnant women
Yellow fever

Diseases in **boldface** should be reported by telephone or telegraph.

*Report number of cases/week.   †Report only if outbreak suspected.

PREVENTING INFECTION AMONG EMPLOYEES

▶ MEDICAL EXAMINATION OF PROSPECTIVE EMPLOYEES

Initial procedures should include:

- Medical history (include immunization history).
- Physical examination.
- Chest X ray.
- VDRL.
- Tuberculin skin test.
- Rubella titer (only for women of childbearing age).

Follow-up should include:

- Skin testing of tuberculin-negative personnel at least once each year.
- (Tuberculin-positive personnel should be checked by an annual chest X ray).
- Necessary immunizations.

Note: The epidemiologic significance of hepatitis B antigenemia is unknown. Routine screening of clinic or hospital employees is not recommended.

▶ TREATMENT OF PERSONNEL WITH ILLNESS

Clinics and hospitals not only have the responsibility of protecting their personnel against acquiring infection from patients, but also the responsibility of protecting patients from acquiring infection from personnel. Thus, all personnel with illness should report to their supervisors or directly to the employee health service. Personnel who have direct or indirect contact with patients via food or fomites should be excused from duty if they have an infection that poses a hazard to patients or to other personnel (e.g., infections of the respiratory tract, the gastrointestinal tract, or the skin).

Personnel who develop infections should be transferred to duties without direct patient contact or should be given sick leave until they are no longer considered hazardous to others. Greater reporting of infectious diseases may be achieved by not penalizing personnel for reporting illness.

Patient care personnel having overt clinical infection, such as streptococcal pharyngitis, acute influenza, or a staphylococcal furuncle, should be restricted from patient contact. Personnel with minor infections can usually continue to work so long as they understand the risk to others and are scrupulous in their practice of personal hygiene (e.g., the nurse or the physician who is recovering from salmonellosis, and who is still excreting salmonellae, usually need not be restricted from patient contact).

Prophylactic therapy should be provided to employees under certain circumstances, such as the use of gamma globulin after intimate exposure to hepatitis A; antibacterial therapy after intimate exposure to meningococcal meningitis (e.g., mouth-to-mouth resuscitation attempts or accidents in the pipetting of spinal fluid); and tetanus toxoid booster immunizations following occupational injuries (if not already immunized).

▶ **IMMUNIZATION OF PERSONNEL**

(See page 218 for standard recommendations, dosages, schedules, and more details.)

Active immunizations

BCG: The use of BCG (bacille Calmette-Guerin) vaccine for tuberculin-negative personnel in patient-contact positions should be considered only in areas serving populations in which the endemic incidence of tuberculosis is high and the hospital employee tuberculin conversion rate is greater than 1% each year for those employed in a specific department or service.

Diphtheria-tetanus: The adult type of combined diphtheria-tetanus (Td) preparation should be given every 10 years, as in the standard recommendations.

Influenza: For those at high risk as in the standard recommendations. Vaccination might be considered for all personnel in anticipation of expected high incidence of influenza.

Measles (rubeola): For nonpregnant women in the childbearing years who are employed in pediatric care and who have not had measles or been immunized.

Mumps: Optional for personnel who have no history of clinical mumps.

Poliomyelitis: For all personnel in accordance with standard recommendations.

Rubella (German measles): For female employees in the childbearing age range who may be exposed to rubella in the line of duty, who are unlikely to become pregnant within 2 months of vaccination, and who demonstrate no antibodies.

Smallpox: Only personnel anticipating contact with patients with smallpox should receive smallpox vaccine.

Passive immunization with immune serum globulin
for exposure to the following:

Hepatitis: Persons who have had parenteral inoculation with needles or instruments contaminated with blood from a patient with hepatitis A or fecal-oral exposure should be given 0.01 ml/kg body weight immune serum globulin (HISG) IM. Hepatitis B immune serum globulin (HBIG) is available on a limited basis.

Smallpox and complications of vaccinia: Special hyperimmune gamma globulin specific for vaccinia and smallpox has been shown to be of value in the management of complications of vaccinations and in modifying disease after exposure.

Varicella–zoster: In accordance with standard recommendations.

▶ **SCREENING CULTURES**

Routine programs designed to detect carriers of pathogens among personnel contribute little to infection control. Programs to detect asymptomatic carriers of staphylococci, streptococci, meningococci, salmonellae, shigellae, and amoebae are not recommended.

▶ **SCREENING CULTURES (Cont.)**

Outbreaks of infections within clinics or hospitals due to such organisms may prompt a search for personnel carriers as part of the study and control of the outbreak.

▶ **EDUCATION PROGRAMS FOR EMPLOYEES**

The broad goals of an education program for any level of employee should:

- Provide an understanding of the basic concepts of infection.
- Provide a working knowledge of the hazards associated with a particular category of employment.
- Convince each employee that he has a personal responsiblity and role in the control of infection within the clinic or hospital.
- Provide a continuing educational program related to infectious disease control.
- Reduce the hazard of acquired infection for each patient and employee.

OUTBREAK INVESTIGATION

▶ **HOW TO INVESTIGATE AN OUTBREAK**

1. *Verify* that there is an outbreak:
   a. Calculate the baseline incidence (endemic) rate of the illness.
   b. Check various sources (such as physicians, hospitals, and schools) to estimate the number of cases.
2. Verify the *diagnosis*:
   a. Be skeptical of unconfirmed information.
   b. Check patients, medical records, laboratory reports.
   c. Confirmation (e.g., by culture) is only needed in severe cases.
3. *Hunt* for additional cases.
   a. Use only several simple, major symptoms (e.g., fever, diarrhea) to identify cases.
   b. Get a rough case-count and establish an attack rate.
4. *Organize* the data by:
   a. *Time*—plot an epidemic curve (see page 248).
   b. *Place*—check distribution by geographic locale, water supply, school districts, etc. Plotting case locations on a map may be useful.
   c. *Person*—check distribution of cases by age, sex, occupation, or other possible risk factor.
5. Develop a hypothesis as to source and mode of transmission.
6. Determine who was or still is at risk.
7. Test the hypothesis by means of statistical analysis of data, surveys, etc.
8. Recommend appropriate control measures.

THE EPIDEMIC CURVE

A simple graph depicting the number of cases of an illness per unit of time may be useful for surveillance purposes or for clearly presenting data from an outbreak. It is customary to represent the number of cases on the vertical scale and time on the horizontal scale.

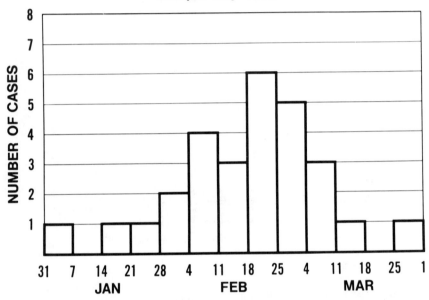

8

EPIDEMIOLOGY—
SOME CONCEPTS AND DEFINITIONS*

CONTENTS
Transmission of Agents Factors Influencing the Spread of Disease Selected Definitions

*Adapted from "Generalizations about Communicable Disease," student material prepared at the University of Pittsburgh, Graduate School of Public Health (unpublished), with material from *Control of Communicable Diseases in Man,* American Public Health Association, Washington, D. C., various editions.

TRANSMISSION OF AGENTS

Modes of transmission are the mechanisms by which an infectious agent is transported from reservoir to susceptible human host. They are contact, airborne, vehicle, and vector.

Contact

- **Direct contact:** Actual touching of the infected person, animal, or other reservoir of infection as in kissing, sexual intercourse, or other contiguous personal association.

- **Indirect contact:** Touching of contaminated objects such as toys, handkerchiefs, soiled clothing, bedding, surgical instruments and dressings, with subsequent hand-to-mouth transfer of infective material; less commonly, transfer to abraded or intact skin or mucous membrane.

- **Droplet spread:** The projection onto the conjunctiva, face, nose, or mouth of the spray emanating from an infected person during sneezing, coughing, singing, or talking. Such droplets usually travel no more than 3 feet from the source. Transmission by droplet infection is considered a form of contact infection, since it involves reasonably close association between two or more persons.

Airborne

Unusual transmission requiring extremely small particles (e.g., smallpox or influenza under special conditions).

Vehicle

Water, food, milk, biologic products (e.g., blood, serum, and plasma) or any substance serving as an intermediate means by which an infectious agent is transported from a reservoir and introduced into a susceptible host through ingestion, through inoculation, or by deposit on skin or mucous membrane.

Vector

Arthropods or other invertebrates that transmit infection by inoculation into or through the skin or mucous membrane by biting, or by deposit of infective materials on the skin or on food or other objects. The vector may be infected itself (e.g., mosquito) or may act only as a mechanical carrier of the agent (e.g., flies' feet carrying shigella).

FACTORS INFLUENCING THE SPREAD OF DISEASE

Characteristics of the organism

Infectivity: Measure of an organism's ability to adapt itself to the environment of the host to the extent of lodging and multiplying. Measure of the least number of organisms capable of producing an infection in a host of a certain species at standard conditions.

Characteristics of the organism (Cont.)

Pathogenicity: Measure of an organism's ability to produce a specific clinical reaction after infection has occurred. Does not refer to the severity of the reaction but to its constancy.

Virulence: Measure of an organism's ability to produce a severe pathologic reaction. Does not refer directly to the regularity of disease production but to its severity once induced.

Toxicity: Measure of an organism's ability to produce a toxic chemical reaction by chemical substances it forms.

Invasiveness: Measure of an organism's ability to penetrate, and extent of distribution after entering a tissue.

Antigenicity: Measure of a microorganism's ability to stimulate an immunologic response in the host.

Characteristics of the host

Resistance-susceptibility: Ability of the host to withstand infection and/or its clinical manifestations. This resistance may be innate or acquired by specific immunologic means.

Immunity: Resistance of a host due to a specific immunologic response (e.g., antibody production). *Passive immunity* usually lasts less than 6 months (e.g., transfer of maternal antibodies across placenta to fetus, artificial inoculation of serum globulin). *Active immunity* usually lasts years (e.g., by natural infection or by artificial inoculaton of killed or modified agents or their toxins).

Infectiousness: Communicability is a measure of the potential ability of an infected host to transmit a disease to other hosts.

Characteristics of the environment

Topographic: The features of a certain location (natural and man-made structures) may affect the occurence and communicability of a specific disease (e.g., histoplasmosis grows well in bat caves).

Geographic: Vector-borne diseases require the geographic presence of the vector.

Sociocultural and/or economic factors (e.g., staphylococcal food poisoning, childhood diarrhea, tuberculosis).

States of communicable disease

The incubation period: This is the interval from the primary invasion to the onset of symptoms. The length depends on the peculiarities of each host-parasite relationship, but the incubation period of a specific infectious disease manifests a constant range of variation. The incubation period may be short when a microparasite has direct access to tissues in which primary multiplication takes place.

States of communicable disease (Cont.)

Clinical manifestations: There is a spectrum or biologic gradient of infections that ranges in severity from inapparent infection to fatal disease. (Subclinical–mild–moderate–severe–fatal.) While a subclinical infection is one without apparent disease, it usually results in an immunologic response.

Carrier states: A carrier is an infected person who harbors a specific infectious agent in the absence of discernible clinical disease, and serves as a potential source of infection for humans. The carrier state may occur with infections inapparent throughout their course (commonly known as healthy carriers), or as a feature of incubation period, convalescence, and postconvalescence of a clinically recognizable disease (commonly known as incubatory and convalescent carriers). Under either circumstance the carrier state may be short or long (temporary or chronic carriers). The same applies to other vertebrate animals.

SELECTED DEFINITIONS

Agent of disease: A substance, infectious or otherwise, that is necessary for the production of specific disease—a *sine qua non* for the disease.

Antiseptic: A chemical compound that stops or inhibits the growth of bacteria without necessarily killing them.

Asepsis: The exclusion of microorganisms causing infection.

Attack rate: A figure reflecting the number of cases of a particular disease or infection in proportion to the total number of individuals at risk during a specified period. For example:

$$\text{Attack rate} = \frac{\text{Number of new infections}}{\text{Number of patients at risk}} \times 100 \quad \text{expressed as } \%$$

Carrier: An infected person who harbors a specific infectious agent without having a discernible clinical disease, and serves as a potential source of infection for others. Carriers with inapparent infections are commonly known as healthy carriers. Carriers in the incubatory or convalescent stage of a clinically recognizable disease are known as incubatory and convalescent carriers. Vertebrate animals other than humans may also be carriers.

Case: Person with disease, usually specifically applied to a diagnosed disease, not an infected person without disease.

Index case: The first case to come to the attention of the investigator. This is not always the primary case.

Primary case: The first case of a communicable disease introduced into the population unit being studied.

Secondary case: Case of disease developing from contact with primary case.

Communicable disease: An illness due to a specific infectious agent or its products that arises through transmission of that agent or its products from a reservoir to a susceptible host; either directly, as from an infected person or animal, or indirectly through the agency of an intermediate plant or animal host, a vector, or the inanimate environment.

Contact: Any person or animal known to have been in such association with an infected person or animal or with a contaminated environment as to have had the opportunity of acquiring the infection.

Contamination: The presence of an infectious agent on a body surface; also on or in clothes, bedding, toys, surgical instruments or dressings, or other inanimate articles or substances including water, milk, and food. Contamination is distinct from pollution, which implies the presence of offensive but noninfectious matter in the environment.

Disinfectant: An agent that destroys or inhibits disease-causing microorganisms.

Disinfection: Killing of infectious agents outside the body by chemical or physical means.

Concurrent disinfection: The application of disinfection as soon as possible after the discharge of infectious material from the body of an infected person, or after the soiling of articles with such infectious discharges, all personal contact with such discharges or articles being prevented prior to such disinfection.

Terminal disinfection: Indicates the process of rendering the personal clothing and immediate physical environment of the patient free from the possibility of conveying the infection to others after the patient has been removed, or has ceased to be a source of infection, or after isolation practices have been discontinued.

Endemic: The habitual presence of a disease within a given geographic area; may also refer to the usual prevalence of a given disease within such area. *Hyperendemic* expresses a persistent activity in excess of expected prevalence.

Endogenous infection: An infection arising from bacteria normally resident in the host.

Epidemic: An epidemic or outbreak is defined as the occurrence in a community or region of a group of illnesses of similar nature, clearly in excess of normal expectancy, and derived from a common or from a propagated source.

Epidemiology: The study of occurrence and distribution of disease.

Exogenous infection: An infection resulting from contamination by a source outside the patient.

Exposure: Circumstances potentially leading to infection.

Fatality rate: Usually expressed as a percentage of the number of persons diagnosed as having a specified disease who die as a result of that illness. The term is frequently applied to a specific outbreak of acute disease in which all patients have been followed for an adequate period of time to include all attributable deaths. The fatality rate must be clearly differentiated from mortality rate. Synonym—fatality percentage.

Fomites: (Singular: fomes.) Any article or substance other than food that may transmit infectious organisms.

Fumigation: Any process by which the killing of animal forms, especially arthropods and rodents, is accomplished by the use of gaseous agents.

Gradient of involvement: Series of gradations of severity from clinically inapparent presence of disease-producing agent through mild, moderate, and severe disease to death. Also called "spectrum" of disease.

Host: A human or other living animal, including birds and arthropods, affording subsistence or lodgment to an infectious agent under natural conditions. Some protozoa and helminths pass successive stages in alternate hosts of different species. Hosts in which the parasite attains maturity or passes its sexual stage are primary or definitive hosts; those in which the parasite is in a larval or asexual state are secondary or intermediate hosts.

Immune person: A person (or animal) that possesses specific protective antibodies or cellular immunity as a result of previous infection or immunization, or is so conditioned by such previous specific experience as to respond adequately with production of antibodies sufficient to prevent clinical illness following exposure to the specific infectious agent of the disease. Immunity is relative; an ordinarily effective protection may be overwhelmed by an excessive dose of the infectious agent or via an unusual portal of entry; may also be impaired by immunosuppressive drug therapy or concurrent disease.

Incidence rate: A quotient (rate), with the number of cases of a specified disease diagnosed or reported during a defined period of time as the numerator, and the number of persons in the population in which they occurred as the denominator. This is usually expressed as cases per 1000 or 100,000/annum. This rate may be expressed as age- or sex-specific or as specific for any other population characteristic or subdivision.

Incubation period: The time interval between exposure to an infectious agent and appearance of the first sign or symptom of the disease in question.

Infected person: A person who harbors an infectious agent and who has either manifest disease or inapparent infection. An infectious person is one from whom the infectious agent can be naturally acquired.

Infection: The entry and development or multiplication of an infectious agent in the body of humans or animals. The presence of living infectious agents on exterior surfaces of the body or upon articles of apparel or soiled articles is not infection but contamination of such surfaces and articles.

Infection chain: Course of transmission from host to host, simple or complicated.
    Homologous infection chain: Transmission from host to host of the same species.
    Heterologous infection chain: Transmission from host of one species to that of another species.

Infectious agent: An organism, chiefly a microorganism but including helminths, that is capable of producing infection or infectious disease.

Infestation: Infestation of persons and animals is the lodgment, development, and reproduction of arthropods on the surface of the body or in the clothing.

Infestation (Cont.)

Infested articles or premises are those which harbor or give shelter to animal forms, especially arthropods and rodents.

Insecticide: Any chemical substance used for the destruction of arthropods, whether applied as powder, liquid, atomized liquid, aerosol, or as a "paint" spray; residual action is usual. The term *larvicide* is generally used to designate insecticides applied specifically for distribution of immature stages of arthropods; *imagocide* or *adulticide* designate those applied to destroy mature or adult forms.

Isolation: The separation for the period of communicability of infected persons from other persons, in such places and under such conditions as will prevent the direct or indirect conveyance of the infectious agent from infected persons to other persons who are susceptible or who may spread the agent to others.

Morbidity rate: An incidence rate used to include all persons in the population under consideration who become ill during the period of time stated.

Mortality rate: A rate calculated in the same way as an incidence rate, using as a numerator the number of deaths occurring in the population during the stated period of time, usually a year. A *total* or *crude* mortality rate utilizes deaths from all causes, usually expressed as deaths per 1000 while a *disease-specific* mortality rate includes only deaths due to one disease and is usually reported on the basis of 100,000 persons.

Nosocomial infection: An infection originating in a medical facility, e.g., occurring in a hospitalized patient in whom it was not present or incubating at the time of admission, or is the residual of an infection acquired during a previous admission. Includes infection acquired in the hospital but appearing after discharge; it also includes infections among staff.

Pathogenicity: The capability of an infectious agent to cause disease in a susceptible host.

Personal hygiene: Those protective measures, primarily within the responsibility of the individual, which promote health and limit the spread of infectious diseases, chiefly those transmitted by direct contact. Such measures encompass (a) keeping the body clean by sufficiently frequent soap and water baths; (b) washing hands in soap and water immediately after voiding bowels or bladder and always before handling food and eating; (c) keeping hands and unclean articles, or articles that have been used for toilet purposes by others, away from the mouth, nose, eyes, ears, genitalia, and wounds; (d) avoiding the use of common or unclean eating utensils, drinking cups, towels, handkerchiefs, combs, hairbrushes, and pipes; (e) avoiding exposure of other persons to spray from the nose and mouth as in coughing, sneezing, laughing, or talking; and (f) washing hands thoroughly after handling a patient or his belongings.

Prevalence rate: A quotient (rate) using as the numerator the number of persons sick or portraying a certain condition, in a stated population, *at a particular time,* regardless of when that illness or condition began, and as the denominator the number of persons in the population in which they occurred. For example, the prevalence rate of ringworm of the foot in a class of boys when examined on a certain day could be 25/100. Or, the prevalence rate of a positive serological test in a survey during which blood samples were collected from a population could be 10/1000.

Quarantine

> *Complete quarantine* is the limitation of freedom of movement of such well persons or domestic animals as have been exposed to a communicable disease, for a period of time equal to the longest usual incubation period of the disease, in such manner as to prevent effective contact with those not so exposed.

> *Modified quarantine* is a selective, partial limitation of freedom of movement of persons or domestic animals, commonly on the basis of known or presumed differences in susceptibility, but sometimes because of danger of disease transmission. It may be designed to meet particular situations; examples are exclusion of children from school or exemption of immune persons from provisions required of susceptible persons, such as contacts acting as food handlers, or restriction of military populations to the post or to quarters.

> *Surveillance* is the practice of close supervision of contacts for purposes of prompt recognition of infection or illness but without restricting their movements.

> *Segregation* is the separation for special consideration, control, or observation of some part of a group of persons or of domestic animals from the others, to facilitate the control of a communicable disease. Examples are: removal of susceptible children to homes of immune persons, or the establishment of a sanitary boundary uninfected from infected portions of a population.

Report of a disease: An official report notifying appropriate authority of the occurrence of a specified communicable or other disease in humans or in animals. Diseases in humans are reported to the local health authority; those in animals to the livestock sanitary or agriculture authority. Some few diseases in animals, also transmissible to humans are reportable to both authorities. Each health jurisdiction declares a list of reportable diseases appropriate to its particular needs. Reports also should list suspect cases of diseases of particular public health importance, ordinarily those requiring epidemiologic investigation or initiation of special control measures.

When a person is infected in one health jurisdiction and the case is reported from another, the authority receiving the report should notify the other jurisdiction, especially when the disease requires examination of contacts for infection, or if food or water or other common vehicles of infection may be involved.

In addition to routine report of cases of specified diseases, special notification is required of all epidemics or outbreaks of disease, including diseases not on the list declared reportable.

Reservoir of infectious agents: Reservoirs are humans, animals, plants, soil, or inanimate organic matter in which an infectious agent lives and multiplies and on which it depends primarily for survival, reproducing itself in such a manner that it can be transmitted to a susceptible host. Humans themselves are the most frequent reservoirs of infectious agents pathogenic for people.

Resistance: The sum total of body mechanisms which interpose barriers to the progress of invasion or multiplication of infectious agents or to damage by their toxic products.

Immunity: That resistance usually associated with possession of antibodies having a specific action of the microorganism concerned with a particular infectious disease or its toxin. *Passive immunity* is attained either naturally by maternal transfer, or artificially by inoculation of specific protective antibodies (convalescent or hyperimmune serum, or immune serum [gamma] globulin [human]); it is of brief duration (days to months). *Active immunity* is attained either naturally by infection with or without clinical manifestations, or artificially by inoculation of fractions or products of the infectious agent or of the agent itself in killed, modified, or variant form. It lasts months to years. Active immunity depends on *cellular immunity* which is conferred by T-lymphocyte sensitization, and *humoral immunity* which is based on B-lymphocyte response.

Inherent resistance: An ability to resist disease independent of antibodies or of specifically-developed tissue response; it commonly resides in anatomic or physiologic characteristics of the host and may be genetic or acquired, permanent or temporary. (Synonym: Nonspecific immunity.)

Rodenticide: A chemical substance used for the destruction of rodents, generally through ingestion.

Source of infection: The person, animal, object, or substance from which an infectious agent passes immediately to a host. Source of infection should be clearly distinguished from source of contamination, such as overflow of a septic tank contaminating water supply, or an infected cook contaminating a salad.

Sterile: Free from microorganisms.

Surveillance of disease: The continuing scrutiny of all aspects of occurrence and spread of disease that are pertinent to effective control. Included are the systematic collection and evaluation of morbidity and mortality reports; of special reports of field investigations, epidemics, and individual cases; of reports of isolations and identifications of infectious agents in laboratories; of data concerning the availability and use of vaccines, immune globulin, insecticides, and other substances used in control; of information regarding immunity levels in segments of the population; and of other relevant epidemiologic data. The procedure applies to all jurisdictional levels of public health, from local to international.

Susceptible: A person or animal presumably not possessing sufficient resistance against a particular pathogenic agent to prevent contracting a disease if or when exposed to the agent.

Suspect: A person whose medical history and symptoms suggest that he may have, or may be developing, some communicable disease.

Transmission of infectious agents: Any mechanism by which a susceptible human host is exposed to an infectious agent. These mechanisms are:

Transmission of infectious agents (Cont.)

Direct transmission: Direct and essentially immediate transfer of infectious agents (other than from an arthropod in which the organism has undergone essential multiplication or development) to a receptive portal of entry through which infection of many may take place. This may be by direct contact as by touching, kissing, or sexual intercourse, or by the direct projection (droplet spread) of droplet spray onto the conjunctiva or onto the mucous membranes of the nose or mouth during sneezing, coughing, spitting, singing, or talking (usually limited to a distance of about 1 meter or less). It may also be by direct exposure of susceptible tissue to an agent in soil, compost, or decaying vegetable matter in which it normally leads a saprophytic existence (e.g., the systemic mycoses) or by the bite of a rabid animal.

Indirect transmission:

Vehicle-borne: Contaminated materials or objects such as toys, handkerchiefs, soiled clothes, bedding, cooking or eating utensils, surgical instruments or dressings (indirect contact); water, food, milk, biological products including serum and plasma; or any substance serving as an intermediate means by which an infectious agent is transported and introduced into a susceptible host through a suitable portal of entry. The agent may or may not have multiplied or developed in or on the vehicle before being introduced into humans.

Vector-borne: (a) *Mechanical*—includes simple mechanical carriage by a crawling or flying insect through soiling of its feet or proboscis, or by passage of organisms through its gastrointestinal tract. This does not require multiplication or development of the organism. (b) *Biological*— Propagation (multiplication), cyclic development, or a combination of these (cyclopropagation) is required before the arthropod can transmit the infective form of the agent to man. An incubation period (extrinsic) is required following infection before the arthropod becomes infective. Transmission may be by saliva during biting, or by regurgitation or deposition on the skin of feces or other material capable of penetrating subsequently through the bite wound or through an area of trauma from scratching or rubbing. This is transmission by an infected nonvertebrate host and must be differentiated for epidemiological purposes from simple mechanical carriage by a vector in the role of a vehicle. An arthropod in either role is termed a vector.

Airborne: The dissemination of microbial aerosols to a suitable portal of entry, usually the respiratory tract. Microbial aerosols are suspensions in the air of particles consisting partially or wholly of microorganisms. Particles in the $1-5$ μ range are easily drawn into the alveoli of the lungs and may be retained there; many are exhaled from the alveoli without deposition.

They may remain suspended in the air for long periods of time, some retaining and others losing infectivity or virulence. Not considered as airborne are droplets and other large particles which promptly settle out.

Transmission of infectious agents (Cont.)

The following are airborne and their mode of transmission is direct:

Droplet nuclei: Usually the small residues which result from evaporation of fluid from droplets emitted by an infected host. Droplet nuclei also may be created purposely by a variety of atomizing devices, or accidentally as in microbiology laboratories or in abattoirs, rendering plants, or autopsy rooms. They usually remain suspended in the air for long periods of time.

Dust: The small particles of widely varying size which may arise from soil (e.g., fungus spores separated from dry soil by wind or mechanical agitation), clothes, bedding, or contaminated floors.

9

QUICK REFERENCE

CONTENTS

ANTIBIOTICS OF CHOICE* (See key on page 264)

	Penicillin	Methicillin-cloxacillin	Ampicillin	Carbenicillin	Cephalosporins	Erythromycin	Tetracycline	Chloramphenicol	Streptomycin	Kanamycin	Gentamicin	Tobramycin	Vancomycin	Polymyxin	Clindamycin	Spectinomycin	Rifampin	Sulfonamides
Gram Negative Bacilli																		
E. coli: urine			S	S	S	R	S	S		S	S	S						S
E. coli: other			1	S	2	R	S	S		S	2	S						
Enterobacter			R	2	R	R		S		1	1	S						
Klebsiella			R	R	1	R	3	3		S	2	S						
Proteus mirabilis			1	S	2	R	R	S		2	1	S						
Proteus (indole pos.)			R	2	R	R	R	R		R	1[a]	S						
Pseudomonas			R	1[a]	R	R	S	R		S	S	S						
Salmonella typhosa			2	S	S	R	S	1		S	S							
Shigella	1		1	S	S	R	S	2		S	S							3
Bacteroides orales		S	S	S	2	S	S	S		R	R				S			
B. fragilis			R	S	2[c]	R	2	1		R	R				1[b]			
Haemophilus influenzae			1				S	S										3
Bordetella pertussis			2			1	2											
Brucella							1	2	2	2	2							
Yersinia pestis (plague)							1[a]	2	1[a]	1	1	S						
Serratia			R	2	R		R	2		R	R			R				

Organism													
Herellea—Mima	R	R	R	R		1	1						2
Cholera	3		R	1	2	2	2				S		
Pasteurella multocida	1	S	2								S	3	
Gram Positive Cocci													
Pneumococci	1		2	2								3	
Streptococcus (beta)	1		2	2									
S. viridans	1^d		2	2									
S. fecalis (**enterococcus**)	2^e	1	3			2^e	S	S					
Microaerophilic streptococci	1		2				S						
Staphylococcus (**coag. pos.**)		1	2	3			S	S	S^g				
Staphylococcus (**coag. neg.**)	2	1	2			3	S	S	2				
Gram Negative Cocci													
Neiseria gonorrheae	1	2	3	2							2		
N. meningitidis	1	3	3	1^f	S								1^f
Gram Positive Bacilli													
Listeria monocytogenes		1		2									
Clostridia perfringens	1		2	2	3							3	
Coryne bacterium diphtheriae	2		1	1	3							3	
Spirochetes													
Treponema pallidum	1		3	2	3								
Leptospira	1		2	2									
Borellia	2		2	1									

(Continued on next page)

ANTIBIOTICS OF CHOICE* (Cont.)

	Penicillin	Methicillin-cloxacillin	Ampicillin	Carbenicillin	Cephalosporins	Erythromycin	Tetracycline	Chloramphenicol	Streptomycin	Kanamycin	Gentamicin	Tobramycin	Vancomycin	Polymyxin	Clindamycin	Spectinomycin	Rifampin	Sulfonamides
Actinomycetes																		
Actinomyces	1					2	2											
Nocardia						2	2[d]									1		1
Miscellaneous																		
Rickettsia							1	2										
Psittacosis							1	2										
Mycoplasma						1	2											
Legionnaires' bac.						1												

1 = First Choice; 2 = Second choice; 3 = Third choice; R = Resistant; S = Sensitive

[a] May be used in combination for synergism.
[b] Given IV.
[c] Cephalosporins ineffective for *Haemophilus influenzae* meningitis; chloramphenicol alternative drug of choice in this situation. (Also true for meningococcal, pneumococcal meningitis.)
[d] Doxycycline, minocycline only.
[e] Combined therapy of gentamicin plus penicillin or cephalosporin.
[f] For carriers only; tetracycline prophylaxis refers to minocycline.
[g] First choice if resistant to methicillin for serious infections.
*Based on sensitivities in Seattle, Washington.

Adapted with permission from: Eisenberg, Mickey and Ray, George C. *Manual of Antimicrobial Therapy and Communicable Diseases.* State of Washington, Department of Social and Health Services, 1976.

CONVERSION FORMULAS AND TABLES

Weight

1 lb = 454 gm, so lb x 454 = gm
1 kg = 2.2 lb, so kg x 2.2 = lb
1 oz = 28 gm
1 grain = 65 mg

CONVERSION OF POUNDS AND OUNCES TO GRAMS

Oz	1 lb	2 lb	3 lb	4 lb	5 lb	6 lb	7 lb	8 lb
				Gm				
0	454	907	1361	1814	2268	2722	3175	3629
1	482	936	1389	1843	2296	2750	3204	3657
2	510	964	1418	1871	2325	2778	3232	3686
3	539	992	1446	1899	2353	2807	3260	3714
4	567	1021	1474	1928	2381	2835	3289	3742
5	595	1049	1503	1956	2410	2863	3317	3771
6	624	1077	1531	1985	2438	2892	3345	3799
7	652	1106	1559	2013	2466	2920	3374	3827
8	680	1134	1588	2041	2495	2948	3402	3856
9	709	1162	1616	2070	2523	2977	3430	3884
10	737	1191	1644	2098	2552	3005	3459	3912
11	765	1219	1673	2126	2580	3033	3487	3941
12	794	1247	1701	2155	2608	3062	3515	3969
13	822	1276	1729	2183	2637	3090	3544	3997
14	851	1304	1758	2211	2665	3119	3572	4026
15	879	1332	1786	2240	2693	3147	3600	4054

Linear measure

1 inch = 2.54 cm
1 foot = 0.3 meters

Volume

1 pint = 500 cc = 16 oz
1 teaspoon = 5 cc

1 tablespoon = 15 cc
1 quart = 0.95 liter

Temperature

(degrees Fahrenheit –32) x 5/9 = degrees Centigrade (Celsius)
(degrees Centigrade x 9/5) + 32 = degrees Fahrenheit

	Centigrade	Fahrenheit	Centigrade	Fahrenheit
	36.0	96.8	38.6	101.4
	36.2	97.1	38.8	101.8
	36.4	97.5	39.0	102.2
	36.6	97.8	39.2	102.5
	36.8	98.2	39.4	102.9
Normal	37.0	98.6	39.6	103.2
range	37.2	98.9	39.8	103.6
	37.4	99.3	40.0	104.0
	37.6	99.6	40.2	104.3
	37.8	100.0	40.4	104.7
	38.0	100.4	40.6	105.1
	38.2	100.7	40.8	105.4
	38.4	101.1	41.0	105.8

REFERENCES

The following references were consulted to verify the summary data presented in this manual. Differences in recommendations between references were at times striking, most notably in such areas as first lines of therapy and drug dosages. Only book references are listed. No attempt was made to document the numerous published articles that helped shape the recommendations outlined in this manual.

A Manual for the Control of Communicable Diseases in California, California State Department of Public Health, 1971.

AMA Drug Evaluation. American Medical Association, 3rd ed., Publishing Sciences Group, Inc., Littleton, Mass., 1977.

Baker, Charles (publisher). *Physicians' Desk Reference* 31st ed. Medical Economics Company, Oradell, N.J., 1977.

Benenson, Abram. *Control of Communicable Diseases in Man*, 12th ed. American Public Health Association, Washington, D.C., 1975.

Brown, H.W. and Belding, D.L. *Basic Clinical Parasitology*, 2nd ed. Appleton-Century-Crofts, New York, 1958.

Dukes, M.M. and Garfield M.N. (Eds.). *Meyler's Side Effects of Drugs by Exerpt Medica.* Volume VIII, American Elsevier Publishing Co., Inc., New York, 1975.

Ibid. Annual Addition, 1977.

Eisenberg, Mickey and Ray, George C. *Manual of Antimicrobical Therapy and Communicable Diseases*, State of Washington, Department of Social and Health Services, 1976.

Facts and Comparisons. Facts and Comparisons, Inc., St. Louis, Mo., 1977 (a monthly-revised update on drug information for pharmacists).

Finland, Maxwell and Kass, Edward H. (Eds.). *Trimethoprim-Sulfamethoxazole-Microbiological, Pharmacological & Clinical Considerations.* University of Chicago Press, Chicago, 1973.

Gardner, Pierce and Provine, Harriet. *Manual of Acute Bacterial Infections*, Little, Brown and Company, Boston, 1975.

Goodman, Louis S. and Gilman, Alfred (Eds.). *The Pharmacological Basis of Therapeutics,* 5th ed. Macmillan Inc., New York, 1975.

Graef, John W. and Cone, Thomas E. (Eds.). *Manual of Pediatric Therapeutics,* 2nd edition, Little, Brown and Company, Boston, 1974.

Hansten, Philip D. (Ed.). *Drug Interactions,* 3rd ed., Lea & Febiger, Philadelphia, 1975.

Headings, Denis L. (Ed.). *The Harriet Lane Handbook,* 7th ed., Year Book Medical Publishers, Inc., Chicago, 1975.

Hirschmann, J. *Infectious Disease Manual,* The Upjohn Company, Kalamazoo, Mich., 1974.

Isolation Techniques for Use in Hospitals, USPHS Publication No. 2054, U.S. Government Printing Office, Washington, 1970.

Kagan, Benjamin M. (Ed.). *Antimicrobial Therapy,* 2nd ed. W. B. Saunders Company, Philadelphia, 1974.

Markell, E.K. and Voge, M. *Medical Parasitology,* 4th ed. W. B. Saunders Company, Philadelphia, 1976.

MMWR, Morbidity and Mortality Weekly Report, Center for Disease Control, USPHS, Vol. 26 (1976), 27 (1977) and part of 28 (1978).

Pratt, William B. (Ed.). *Chemotherapy of Infection*, Oxford University Press, Inc., New York, 1977.

Report of the Committee on Infectious Diseases, 17th ed., American Academy of Pediatrics, AAP, 1974.

Shirkey, Harry (Ed.). *Pediatric Drug Handbook.* W. B. Saunders Company, Philadelphia, 1977.

The Medical Letter, Vol. 16 (1974), 17 (1975), 18 (1976), 19 (1977) and part of 20 (1978). The Medical Letter, Inc., New Rochelle, N. Y.

Thorn, George, *et al. Harrison's Principles of Internal Medicine,* 8th ed., McGraw-Hill Book Company, 1977.

INDEX

Pages in bold type indicate main discussion of disease or drug.